The Lucky Ones

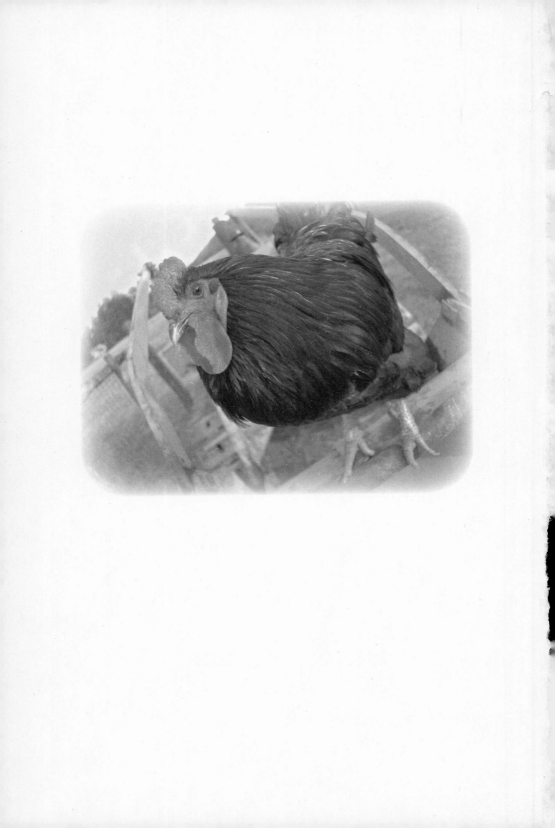

The Lucky Ones

My Passionate Fight for Farmed Animals

Jenny Brown

Founder, Woodstock Farm Animal Sanctuary

with Gretchen Primack

AVERY

a member of Penguin Group (USA) Inc.

New York

Published by the Penguin Group
Penguin Group (USA) Inc., 375 Hudson Street, New York, New York 10014,
USA • Penguin Group (Canada), 90 Eglinton Avenue East, Suite 700, Toronto, Ontario
M4P 2Y3, Canada (a division of Pearson Penguin Canada Inc.) • Penguin Books Ltd, 80 Strand,
London WC2R 0RL, England • Penguin Ireland, 25 St Stephen's Green, Dublin 2, Ireland (a division
of Penguin Books Ltd) • Penguin Group (Australia), 250 Camberwell Road, Camberwell, Victoria
3124, Australia (a division of Pearson Australia Group Pty Ltd) • Penguin Books India Pvt Ltd,
11 Community Centre, Panchsheel Park, New Delhi–110 017, India • Penguin Group (NZ), 67 Apollo
Drive, Rosedale, North Shore 0632, New Zealand (a division of Pearson New Zealand Ltd) • Penguin
Books (South Africa) (Pty) Ltd, 24 Sturdee Avenue, Rosebank, Johannesburg 2196, South Africa

Penguin Books Ltd, Registered Offices: 80 Strand, London WC2R 0RL, England

Recipes

Page 248, Insanely Tasty *VegNews* Mac 'n' Cheese: Colleen Holland (originally published in
VegNews magazine); page 250, Quick Savory Nut Loaf: Adapted from *The Complete Vegetarian
Cuisine* by Rose Elliot, Pantheon Books, New York; page 252, Almond Feta Cheese with Herb Oil:
Rochelle Palermo, from *Vegetarian Times*, April 2009; page 254, Cashew Pumpkin Tartlets: Pamela
Brown; p.255, Speedy yet Heavenly Thai Basil Sesame Noodles: People for the Ethical Treatment of
Animals, www.peta.org; page 258, Blueberry-Lemon Corn Biscuit Cobbler: Excerpted from *Vegan
Pie in the Sky: 75 Out-of-This World Recipes for Pies, Tarts, Cobblers, and More*, by Isa Chandra
Moskowitz and Terry Hope Romero (Da Capo Lifelong, 2011).

Most Avery books are available at special quantity discounts for bulk purchase for sales promotions,
premiums, fund-raising, and educational needs. Special books or book excerpts also can be
created to fit specific needs. For details, write Penguin Group (USA) Inc.
Special Markets, 375 Hudson Street, New York, NY 10014.

Library of Congress Cataloging-in-Publication Data
Brown, Jenny.
The lucky ones : my passionate fight for farm animals / Jenny Brown with Gretchen Primack.
p.   cm.
Includes bibliographical references and index.
ISBN 978-1-58333-441-6
1. Brown, Jenny.   2. Woodstock Farm Animal Sanctuary.   3. Animal sanctuaries—New York (State)—Woodstock.
4. Domestic animals—New York (State)—Woodstock.   5. Animal rights activists—United States—Biography.
6. Animal welfare—Moral and ethical aspects—United States.   7. Brown, Jenny—Childhood.   8. Cancer in
children—Patients—United States—Biography.   9. Bones—Cancer—Patients—United States—Biography.
I. Primack, Gretchen.   II. Title.
HV4716.B76A3   2012   2012010041
636.08'32092—dc23
[B]

Printed in the United States of America
1 3 5 7 9 10 8 6 4 2

BOOK DESIGN BY NICOLE LAROCHE

The recipes contained in this book are to be followed exactly as written. The publisher is not responsible for your
specific health or allergy needs that may require medical supervision. The publisher is not responsible for any adverse
reactions to the recipes contained in this book.

While the authors have made every effort to provide accurate telephone numbers and Internet addresses at the time of
publication, neither the publisher nor the authors assume any responsibility for errors, or for changes that occur after
publication. Further, the publisher does not have any control over and does not assume any responsibility for author or
third-party websites or their content.

Penguin is committed to publishing works of quality and integrity. In that spirit, we are proud to offer this book to our
readers; however, the story, the experiences, and the words are the authors' alone.

To my incredible husband, Doug,
the love of my life, for making all I do possible,
and for his infinite support, love, patience,
and humor. He's a keeper!

In memory of Julie Goodloe

I am the voice of the voiceless;
Through me the dumb shall speak,
Till the deaf world's ear be made to hear
The cry of the wordless weak.
From street, from cage and from kennel,
From jungle and stall, the wail
Of my tortured kin proclaim the sin
Of the mighty against the frail.

—Ella Wheeler Wilcox (1850–1919),
"The Voice of the Voiceless"

Contents

Prologue

I t's Saturday morning, and I'm in Mission Control. That's what
I call my office, which is on the second story of my house and
has a glorious view of the entire farm. Through the windows
behind my computer, I see three white turkeys, Petunia, Beatrice,
and Sphinx, pecking leftover grain in the grass. Farther out,
2,000-pound Andy the steer is tossing a pine branch up in the air
with his horns—pine needles are like catnip for cows. Half a dozen
goats of various sizes are playing King of the Rock Pile. Rod the
rooster humps a volunteer's shoe (he's got a foot fetish), which
cracks me up as usual. The bunnies are just a blur as they dart in
and out of their habitat. Arnell the goose is honking his usual false
alarm over something innocuous. Now you know why I don't need
HBO.

This is Woodstock Farm Animal Sanctuary. My husband, Doug,
and I, along with our small staff and volunteers, take care of
around two hundred farm animals. They are all rescues, and they
all will get to live out their natural lives in peace.

Prologue

But it's not all entertaining: I watch our farm manager, Sheila, lead a young sheep named Summer slowly out of her barn. Summer's got an appointment four hours away at Cornell Veterinary Hospital to have her recently weakened back end X-rayed, and the whole farm is worried sick about her. Riding shotgun with Sheila will be Bruce, a rooster whose infected foot isn't healing with the usual methods. Stubby the pig is also doing poorly, and we expect a similar journey soon. We drive the four hours because vets with extensive knowledge of farm animals are few and far between. The typical farmer would simply cull the animal, the thought of a vet visit never entering his mind.

Coco, a blind chicken who shares my office, walks over and cozies up to my foot. From the looks of the blanket on the floor, she's just laid an egg, and the effort of creating a nest and laying the egg wears her out and makes her sleepy. I lean down to give her neck a stroke, and then I catch a glimpse of a car full of visitors cruising up our long gravel drive. The sanctuary's open to the public on the weekends for farm tours, and pretty soon our modest visitors' center will be filled with people curious about what we do and eager to get close to animals. I love to connect visitors to the residents of Woodstock Farm Animal Sanctuary, WFAS for short, and it's a good thing I do, since that's how I'm going to spend the day. I tap on Coco's feed bowl and she perks up, using various sounds in my office to orient herself. Then I get ready to go outside.

By the time I arrive at the picnic tables, a dozen people—families, couples, and a lone figure or two—are waiting for me. They look around at our pastures, barns, and coops, all set against a backdrop of the green Catskill Mountains. I greet the group and tell them a little about how this crazy idea became a reality. But before I can finish the thought, a tall turkey ambles on over, feathers white against his crazy red head. "This is Boone, our friendliest, most outgoing turkey," I say, kneeling down and smoothing down his feathers. "You've probably all heard that turkeys are too dumb to get out of the rain, or that they will actually drown in the rain? Well, that's an urban legend. These guys are as smart and personable as the cats and dogs you may have at home."

We walk on the gravel path past the inquisitive goats and a couple of roaming chickens, and I start to explain the history of factory farming, how it really took off after World War II. The group is my captive audience: They'll get to have lots of fun meeting our residents, but the "price" they pay is that I'm not going to sugarcoat the important information I want them to hear.

By now, we've reached the barn that Boone and other turkeys share with the pigs, a few of whom are snoring on their sides out in the sun. "Come say hello to these guys," I urge the group. There are a couple of nervous laughs and gasps, and I understand. These are no little potbellies; they are each easily seven or eight hundred pounds.

I push through the gate and kneel in the straw next to a half-awake Louie, who stretches his snout in one direction and his hooves in the other when he feels my hand scratch his belly. His bliss is so obvious and sweet that the visitors follow me one by one. A kid on the tour reaches out and barely touches Louie before jerking his hand back with a laugh. The next time he touches him, though, he gently smoothes his bristly hair. Soon he is stroking him like a dog.

That's when I start talking about the difference in the lives of all of Louie's less lucky brothers, born into an industrialized system with only two goals: fast and cheap. I'm not exaggerating too much when I call them brothers; modern breeding sows are artificially inseminated and the gene pool is deliberately kept small to provide a uniform "product."

People start asking the usual great questions. Why do pigs like to roll in the mud? Do chickens require a rooster to be present to lay eggs? Why do some cows have horns? Do ducks mate for life? Where do you get your animals? What's up with the eyes of goats being so odd-looking? Between questions, I tell the visitors each animal's story and more about individual personalities.

I tell them how devoted sister pigs Patsy and Judy are to each other, and, just like human sisters, how incredibly snotty they can be to each other. I tell them how Elvis the steer cries with loneliness if any of his bovine buddies go to the vet. How Louise the sheep will look you deep in the eyes and then press her head against your hip, demanding affection as if her life depended on it. How Mickey the duck will wrap his wing completely around his girlfriend Jo on a winter day, protecting her from the chill and the amorous intentions of others.

I also show them actual models of cages and crates, and talk to them about what's missing from our collective understanding of meat, eggs, dairy, down feathers, and wool. On the surface this seems like just so much chitchat, charming stories interspersed with healthy doses of reality and buzzkill, but something very important is happening. Whether through a major epiphany or a tiny little synapse firing, nobody leaves the farm without being changed in some way.

That's why I do what I do, and it took me only thirty-two years to figure it out.

The Cat and the Cripple

Running a sanctuary involves many firsts—the first time a hen caged her whole life is allowed to stretch her wings, the first time a pig tries an apple, the first time two goats destined to be best friends meet, and so on. Little Dylan was a first, too: our first newborn. By the time he came to us, I had cared for plenty of young to ancient farm animals. Trimming pig hooves, vaccinating goats, treating bumblefoot on turkeys, administering injectable parasite treatments—these were all in a day's filthy, happy, and sometimes harrowing work. But now there was someone brand new, literally, at our sanctuary: an anxious calf all of five days old, a sweet lil' Holstein boy with spindly legs, huge brown eyes, and a tongue that could wrap itself around your whole hand with one lick.

Dylan, who we'd named after the musical god himself—we were in Woodstock, after all—had spent the first four of those five days tied to a tree on a small dairy farm in Troy, New York. Newborn calves like Dylan are taken from their mothers quickly, usually within one to three days. The farmer makes his money per gallon of milk, so allowing the calves to drink it (never mind that it was intended for them) is a waste of profits. Instead, farmers give the calves a cheap powdered milk replacer that's laden with antibiotics to keep them from getting sick from stress. The girls are moved to another facility away from the mothers who they will eventually replace in the herd, and the males are sold off very young for meat, usually to veal farmers. Dylan was unwillingly waiting for just such a farmer as he stood tied to that tree. He was lucky, though. A caring couple saw him there, managed to strike a deal with the farmer, and took him home to save his life. But the next day, feeling overwhelmed, they called our fledgling sanctuary and asked if we could take him in.

Now here he was, stressed and confused but curious—and ridiculously cute. Seriously: In the realm of cuteness, few could be higher on the throne than this little guy. I took a deep breath and looked at my husband, Doug, who was taking a deep breath, too. Then we knelt down to meet him, his giant pink nose meeting my face. He sniffed my head and licked my hair, leaving a tendril of slobbery goo.

To keep him warm and comfy, we decided to set Dylan up in a spacious pen in the pigs' barn. We laid out heaps of fluffy straw for him to lie on and hay for him to snack on. Sophie and Pig-Pig, two older motherly sows, came over to check out the new arrival through the boards surrounding his pen, sniffing and making their friendly grunts at the baby. It's no wonder he brought out their maternal instinct—hell, he'd have brought out the maternal instinct in a heavyweight boxer.

I stared at Dylan and thought about how lucky he was to

escape his fate. If he'd been trucked over to the veal farm he was intended for, he would have been shoved into a narrow stall and chained by the neck. There he would have stayed, day after day, and would not have stepped out of it again until he was slaughtered. In the six months leading up to that day, he would be fed an iron-poor, drug-laced liquid diet in order to create the pale, anemic flesh that typifies veal. Such confinement and isolation is misery for any animal, but on top of that he would be suffering from painful diarrhea caused by stress, bacteria, and anemia. This is the grim fate of the veal calf, a by-product of the dairy industry. Tears of relief came to my eyes as I thanked the powers that be for leading him to us. One thing I knew for sure: Dylan would never end up on someone's fork.

Olivia, a white goat about ten years old, glanced over at the new baby with her trademark look of total indifference. Every so often, her long, velvety ears would twitch with interest and her dark eyes would fix on Dylan, but then she'd walk a couple of feet away and graze a bit, as if to say, "He isn't *that* interesting. . . ."

Olivia was a fellow resident of the pig barn who'd been with us for just a few weeks. Her owners had abandoned her in a rickety barn when their house burned down. Her hooves had grown so long they contorted her legs and made walking difficult and painful. She had spent weeks standing around alone, drinking from a mud puddle and sniffing in vain for something to eat. A compassionate neighbor was good enough to provide food for her and reach out to a wildlife rehabber, who took one look at her and called us.

Olivia was our very first rescued goat, and when she arrived, she was scared and very on guard. She didn't want to be touched. She'd butt me with her horns or snap at my hand if I reached out to her.

She was underweight and her coat, infested with mites, was mangy and dull.

But as time passed, the hoof trimming, liniment rubs on her knobby knees, high-quality grain, and hay and vitamin supplements, as well as equal amounts of treats, attention, and love, were working wonders. Olivia liked to be around people now, and allowed us to pet her lovely creamy coat. She'd escort us on our rounds all day, enjoying her freedom and her caretaker friends. But she still had little use for any of the other animals on the farm.

I decided to indulge her for a moment before going back in with Dylan, so I played "the butt" game with her. This meant pushing my hands against her Princess Leia horns and watching her jump in the air, land, and gently push or butt back again. After a few minutes playing, Doug led her back outside to graze, and I went in to get to know little Dylan.

Dylan stood on his spindles and looked up at me. When I reached a hand forward to pet him, he immediately tried to suckle my fingers. The poor little guy: The most natural thing in the world for him at that age would have been to be with his mother night and day, nursing whenever he wanted to, nuzzling and being nuzzled, and never leaving her side. Instead, he'd been torn from her and left alone and confused.

I fantasized about going to the farmer and pleading for Dylan's mother, but I knew that would be a losing fight. The farmer would never have given her up: To him, she was a moneymaking milk machine, and eventually she would be sold and slaughtered for hamburger. Ground beef often comes from the worn-out, battered bodies of dairy cows who are sent to the slaughterhouse around four years of age when milk production declines. Those commodities are too precious to give up to some romantic notion of mother-son love. The farmer wouldn't even recognize that love, wouldn't permit it in his mind; that way, he feels no guilt for his work. In any case, we don't believe in buying animals to save them, as much as I would like to. Putting money in those pockets means we become part of the problem. He'd just turn around and use our funds to buy two or three scared little girl calves, themselves torn away from their own mothers, to start the cycle over again. Still, I know animals saved from a horrifying death could care less how the rescue happened. I think of that often. I would want to be bought if it would save my life. Their lives are as precious to them as ours are to us.

■ ■ ■ ■

As soon as I knew we'd be taking in Dylan, I called knowledgeable friends, hit the books, and hopped on the Internet to research his care. How often should he be fed? What should I look for as signs of illness? What vaccinations were recommended? I felt like I'd just adopted a child, suddenly looking responsibility and commitment in the face—admittedly, an insanely sweet face with a big pink, velvety nose. He became our responsibility every bit as much as a human child would have, and I took that duty very seriously. It is, after all, a life.

And now here I was, about to give him his first feeding. I readied a two-liter bottle of milk replacer and stood beside him in his pen, hopeful that the suckling would calm him. But what I thought would be a sweet, gentle, memorable moment turned out to be me holding on for dear life as his powerful sucking action almost ripped the bottle out of my hands. It took all I had to hold the bottle still and keep the nipple in his mouth. Talk about excitement! His tail spun around like a lopsided propeller, as he pushed and sucked with all his might. And just like that, the milk was gone.

Looking for more, he rooted and pushed against my belly, my hip, and then my butt, smearing all my clothes with milky drool. When he realized there wasn't any more, he started frolicking, skinny legs tangling up. I rolled a big red rubber ball over to him, a horse toy the pigs loved to play with. He wobbled over to snuffle it, cocking his head with curiosity, and in so doing he accidentally moved it forward. Whoa—the game was on! I kicked it outside, and he ran after the ball, stumbling over it with his top-heavy body, kicking his back legs in the air. As soon as that moment came, it was gone again, just as it would be with a child. He lost interest completely. Realizing that his belly was full, his eyes now heavy, he knelt down, front knees then back, and curled his legs underneath himself. He squeezed his eyes shut and rubbed his face in the deep grass, then passed out.

I can't think of anything that makes me happier than seeing an animal's contentment, witnessing a creature allowed to be who he wants to be in the world—and at peace. It's a thing of beauty. I could feel the anxiety drain out of me as I watched Dylan sleep in the sunlight. For a while, I just sat with him, deeply content myself, and I realized that I must have been feeling some form of maternal love. Doug and I know that our lives are too busy, our personal finances too limited, our passion for our cause too strong to ever have children of our own. When I turned forty, I kept wondering whether I would regret this decision, but to put more bodies on a planet that can't sustain the ones already on it just didn't make sense. And who's to say our offspring, despite our best efforts, might not turn out to be, well, an asshole? Like the next Ted Nugent—my worst nightmare! I guess in the future we could always adopt, or as Doug calls it, "recycle." In the meantime, I realized that I DO have children whom I love as my own; they just happen to all have fur or feathers.

That evening, when Doug and I left Dylan nestled in his warm, straw-filled pen, he let out high-pitched moos of protest. I knew I couldn't just go off to bed and leave him out there in the barn. Not an option. I grabbed a sleeping bag from the house and brought it out to the barn, then fluffed up some straw underneath it and crawled in. Dylan sniffed me and immediately quieted. It took him almost no time to fall asleep, but I lay awake listening to the night sounds of the barn. On one side of us slept twelve pigs, shifting, snorting, and farting—loudly. On the other side, Olivia was curled up like a furry, softly snoozing snowball, and a few free-roaming chickens who also slept in the pig barn were waking and clucking at the erupting pig farts. It wasn't the first time I'd spent the night with a farm animal, nor would it be the last. But it was my first overnight in the pig barn, and I enjoyed the experience. Doug, more partial to thread count than straw bale, gracefully bowed out.

At rooster-crow time the next morning when I opened my eyes, I saw Dylan craning his neck to try to lick Olivia, who was calmly chewing her cud over in the next pen. She was totally ignoring him, like she ignored the other animals on the farm when they'd try to sniff her or beckon her over to their fences with moos and neck stretches. Dylan seemed so earnest, though, I held out hope that the little guy would win her over.

Dawn, our friend and a new board member at the time, slept

with Dylan the next night to help get him acclimated to his new home. Everyone loved taking turns giving him his bottle. When time permitted, we'd gather around to watch the spectacle. We also started him on small amounts of grain to help put weight on him going into the winter. We learned quickly, though, that Dylan was crafty and could nose the lid open on the can of grain that sat next to his pen. His tummy ache alerted us to that one. And, indeed, though it's common practice for factory farmers to fatten their cows with grain, ruminants aren't designed to digest it beyond small amounts—it can lead to awful cramps and gas; at worst, it's lethal. As soon as we saw how sneaky Dylan was about getting into the can, we designed a gated pen to store the open bags of feed. It was just too tempting for a free-roaming, people-following calf.

A few evenings after Dylan came to live with us, as we were closing up the farm for the night, I poked my head into the barn, and I thought my heart would explode. Dylan and Olivia were pressed against each other, as close as they could be on either side of the pen door that separated them. We cracked the gate and invited Olivia into Dylan's pen, and she walked right over to him, stretching her neck to get a good sniff. He nuzzled and licked her, and she let him, standing still and closing her eyes. Doug and I were blown away by the quick transition from resident curmudgeon to surrogate mom.

From that morning on, amazingly, Dylan and Olivia grazed together, slept together, and kinda sorta played together. Dylan was a frisky boy to say the least. With his buddy and goat mom by his side, his joy would manifest in crazy bouts of running in circles and bucking and butting. At first, he was small enough that we didn't worry much. There they'd be, each in a fuzzy fleece jacket against the November chill, Olivia lowering those Princess Leia horns and Dylan kicking up those skinny legs. Sometimes his excitement would lead to sideways-bucking freak-outs, and you could almost see her rolling her eyes. If he got too close, she would swing her head at him, and he'd take a couple steps back and keep kicking up his legs in a circle around her. She'd graze, relaxed, and soon enough he'd calm down and follow suit, ripping up huge mouthfuls of sweet grass. It was unconditional love on his part and a cocktail of maternal instincts and tolerance on hers, which, I suppose, is what motherhood is all about.

But as he grew—and he grew fast!—we kept a careful eye on them together. At one point they were the same size. By six months, he was as big as a pony. By a year, he was close to eight hundred pounds. They were both getting older, and while for Dylan that meant growing up, for Olivia it meant growing old. Her face became gaunter, her backbone more pronounced, and her legs grew knobby and frail. One day, in an especially lively moment, Dylan nuzzled his friend right onto her side. After that, tough as it was to do, the safest thing was to have him spend his daytime hours with the other three steer. They welcomed him, licking him all over, but he still looked for his "mom," pacing the fence and mooing loudly. Once his energy waned in the evenings, we felt comfortable leading him back to the barn to sleep with Olivia, but we just couldn't risk an unintentional injury to her during playtime.

Eventually, Dylan grew so big that he stayed day and night with his steer brothers. But he and Olivia could always be seen grazing or lying down chewing their cud with their bodies pressed against each other through the woven wire.

The Lucky Ones

....

When I watch Dylan play—and I still do, all 2,000 pounds of him—I see the dog in him, the cat, the boy. For me and many others who share my philosophy about animals, species doesn't matter. We're all on a level playing field, none more important than another. Animals are here with us, not *for* us—that's my motto. All of the animals I live with, from our dog Carli to our rooster Rod, want the same things: companionship, pleasure, good food, room to explore, and the freedom to spend their days as they wish. When sheep Ruby Bird or Ashton use a hoof to paw at your leg for attention, it's just like Carli, who has been known to scratch the skin off a shin. When Rod stretches his wings in the sun and lies down to sunbathe, he reminds me of our cat Pogo, who stretches his front paws in the sun, flops over on his side, and goes to sleep. Andy the steer, who also escaped his fate as veal chops, trots over when he's called, just like a dog. And Ophelia the hen, whose wings and thighs would have ended up on a plate, just wants to crawl into your lap to snuggle and mooch your warmth—just like a cat.

Their faces may not express emotions the same way ours do, but it's hard to miss bliss when you see it.

When I was little, my only connection to the animal world was, like most American children, cats and dogs, along with a few squirrels and the sad hostages at the zoo. When I was ten, I finally got the pet I'd been begging for since I left the womb, a tiny calico wisp of a kitten with huge orange spots. At that time, I felt the world owed me something and that I was therefore justified in asking for whatever I wanted. Hobbling around bald and gaunt, dangling a severed limb, can make you feel that way.

The sad reason I'd finally won the battle to have a pet is that I'd been diagnosed with bone cancer. I had already had my leg amputated and begun my long course of chemotherapy treatments. I felt isolated by my illness; sure, I had my mom, sister, grandparents, and friends, but they had full lives outside my sickroom. I wanted a steadfast companion. Someone who could be there when I needed—and someone who was oblivious to what I was going through. I wanted a pet.

Before I was diagnosed, I was as active as a kid could be. I used that right leg for cartwheel after cartwheel, for sprinting around the bases, to swim, dance, and take my beloved gymnastic classes. It braced me when I pushed back the coffee table in my grandparents' house for one of my frequent impromptu contemporary dance recitals, or to chase the boys in school and run around my south end of Louisville neighborhood with abandon.

But a few months after my tenth birthday and months of debilitating chemotherapy treatments, my doctor came into my hospital room in the children's cancer ward. The look on his face wasn't heartening. I could feel my throat close before he even took a breath.

"Jenny, we were hoping that the drugs we've been giving you would kill the tumor," he said, sitting down across from me, "but instead the disease is spreading faster than we can treat it."

I managed to take a breath. "But you're not going to cut my leg off like Sam's, right?" Samantha was a sixteen-year-old on my ward. She'd sit in the visitors' waiting area and chain-smoke (that was back when people were allowed to light up in hospitals—nuts!).

"I'm sorry, but that's the only option. If we don't remove the leg," he said in his strong Indian accent, "the cancer could spread and kill you."

I turned to my mom. "You're not going to let them do that, Mommy, are you?"

"Jenny, you'll die otherwise—we have to." She pressed a tissue to her nose, her eyes swollen.

"No! You can't let them! They want to *chop* my *leg* off!! Don't I have a say?! It's MY leg!" I wailed. "I'd rather die!"

And I meant it. I was more terrified by the prospect of losing part of my body than I had been, just a few months before, when I learned that I had cancer. I had already dealt with losing all of my hair from the chemo, and the treatments made me violently ill. I didn't think it could be worse until now. The specter of someone hacking off my limb, of becoming a "cripple" at age ten, an amputee, was straight out of a horror film. I tried to picture myself with a stump where my leg had been, but I couldn't: Terror shut the image down. My only consolation was an irrational, childish belief that the leg would somehow grow back. I'd seen that happen in a late-night movie, *Swamp Thing*, so I genuinely thought it could happen to me, until my mother burst that bubble.

My religious mother had her own coping mechanism: her faith. Our family went to church three times a week without fail. Mom was moved and strengthened when my grandfather came to the hospital, the night before my surgery, with his fellow deacons and our pastor. A dozen men surrounded my hospital bed to pray for me. They were dressed for the occasion, in suits and wide ties, hair carefully combed back, the smell of Vitalis fighting the usual odor of disinfectant. One deacon prayed aloud with his eyes to heaven, fluorescent light flashing off his horn-rimmed glasses, while the others bowed their heads.

"In the Name of the Father, of the Son Jesus Christ, and by the power of the Holy Spirit, I set this oil apart to be the Holy Anointing Oil," intoned the leader, and touched my forehead with his oily thumb. He made the sign of the cross as he continued, "Through this holy anointing may the Lord in his love and mercy help you with the grace of the Holy Spirit. May the Lord who frees you from sin save you and raise you up." And the men chorused, "Amen!"

As comforting as it was supposed to be, the fact that these grown men took the time to gather in solemn prayer and somber mood around me made me wonder if they and my doctors were keeping me in the dark. "I could die," I thought as they prayed. Or something else terrible could happen. Tears soaked my blanket as I lay there thinking for the first time that having my leg cut off might not be the cure: I had to go through this horrible thing without the assurance that I would even beat the cancer. Would I lose both legs? Both arms? My life? People died all the time in hospitals on TV.

I said good-bye to my leg on a fall day, the perfect kind Louisville gave us every year. It was a day I should have spent running through the backyard and rolling in the leaves, both feet poking through the raked piles. Instead, I was having my leg scoured and sanitized by hospital staff.

Just before surgery, I had a final moment with my whole body. I looked down at my leg, shiny and swollen and stained orange with iodine, as the nurse pushed something into my IV line and began wheeling me down to the surgical floor. The sedative and my tears made the ride surreal and blurry, like a strange dream or, rather, a nightmare. Then the wheels of the gurney were locked with a jolt. A plastic mask lowered onto my face. I began counting down life as I had known it, and then I was out.

When I regained consciousness, I was alone in a dim room. It took a few minutes for my head to clear enough to remember what had happened, but even in my groggy state I could feel an intense, unrelenting pain in my leg. Not just at my knee, but all the way down to my heel and toes. Amid the incredible pain I felt relief—sure it hurt, but they must have found a way to save the leg—I could feel it! While I was under, they must have discovered that all the cancer could be removed without amputation. Could it be? High on pain meds and still woozy from anesthesia, I somehow managed to prop up on my elbows just high enough to see my left leg under the sheet. Then my eyes traveled over to the right. Below the lump of my knee, all I saw was flat expanse.

I screamed. I screamed until my throat felt grated, so loudly that my mother heard me down the hall in the waiting room, that nurses came running from their station, calling my name.

The next few weeks were saturated in pain—some of it, as they'd warned me but I hadn't grasped, phantom pain. They had severed my bone a few inches below the knee, and then wrapped my calf muscle up under the remaining bone to serve as padding for the stump. My body was protesting this radical repositioning, every second of every minute of every hour. The stump was swaddled in bandages that had to be changed daily; meanwhile, even the slightest movement caused excruciating pain. I was on morphine and Demerol and always begging for more, a ten-year-old junkie. And my anger and sense of loss—loss of a limb and of a normal life—ran as deep as the pain.

Meanwhile, my leg was off doing the traveling I'd never done. I'd hardly left Kentucky, but portions of my bone jetted off to California and New York for tumor study. I had wanted to keep my severed leg: If I couldn't have it attached to me anymore, at least I could preserve it in Plexiglas, which somehow seemed reasonable to me at the time (though repulsive to others). But the decision and arrangements had been made—like all of these life-changing ones—without me.

My nurses thought I was the worst kid they'd ever dealt with, and I don't blame them. They'd come into my room and I'd call them everything I could think of, hollering and wailing before they'd even touched me. I'd scream profanities. My mother would try to calm me down and I'd scream at her. Another nurse would come in a few hours later to rotate me to stave off bedsores—more pain, more shrieking, more throwing things, more spinning my head around like Regan in *The Exorcist*. I couldn't have imagined worse pain; that is, until one day a doctor came in to remove the drainage tube that had been inserted in my leg, just above the amputation. He ripped it out in one go. I almost passed out.

My mother was stalwart, and Lord knows how she was able to handle the hellion her daughter had become. I'm sure her faith helped her, but it didn't feel like God was helping me. It's not that I was giving up on God—that didn't feel like an option, considering my upbringing, no matter what I was going through. Southern Baptism focuses a lot on judgment, so I thought this cancer thing might have been punishment. Was it all the fighting with my sister? Disobedience to my mother or grandparents? The make-out sessions with my fourth-grade boyfriend? Or maybe it wasn't something we mortals could understand, since I kept hearing, "God has a plan." But if God did have a plan, how did mine end up being so terrible? I believed Jesus knew if I acted up, but I couldn't control my temper tantrums. Jesus was like Santa Claus, keeping track of who's naughty or nice. I only hoped I could play the cancer card and change columns in his list.

When the hospital psychologist chastised me for my rude and disrespectful behavior, I couldn't believe it. Did he live in some other universe, some endlessly cheerful and polite *Leave It to Beaver* world? My life as I knew it had been taken from me—my identity, my health, my looks, my sense of humor, my friends, my confidence, my childhood. What was this guy smoking? Of course I was pissed off at the world. Even the act of thinking was almost impossible in such a drugged state; every decision seemed out of my hands. Worse, everyone else was going about living their lives and I was a gaunt, jaundiced, emaciated kid with half a leg and a bald head who was spending way too much time in a hospital bed. I had no one to relate to, no one who could even imagine this. The other sick children were always rotating in and out of the ward and were often too ill to befriend or even bond with casually, as kids often do. I was lonely and scared, a victim, and I acted the part with flair.

I took my anger out on my mother as much as anyone, but I also craved her comfort. She had a grueling schedule working nights as an obstetrics nurse in that same hospital. In the morning, after her shift, instead of going home to a quiet apartment for some quality sleep, she would come up two flights and crawl into my twin hospital bed.

"You awake?" she'd whisper as she slipped off her shoes. "Were you up a lot last night?"

"I was sick just after midnight," I told her. "I hit the nurse button and had to ask for more Phenergan."

"I'm sorry, baby girl," she sighed. "Do you feel like eating anything?"

"No, just climb in bed with me, please!"

If she slept at all, she did it right there throughout my recuperation. While we were awake, she spent every extra moment trying to get me to eat, knitting caps for my bald head, playing games and reading with me, buying me whatever junk food and toys she could afford, inching along behind me with my IV pole as I learned how to walk with crutches, the pain still agonizing.

Even though my leg was a goner, the doctors were concerned that a renegade cell may have spread beyond the leg, so I was looking at eighteen more months of chemo. Thanks to my mother's nursing skills, I was able to move home and do two out of three chemo treatments as an outpatient. This meant more time outside Kosair Children's Hospital, and that meant interacting with people who weren't used to seeing sick kids. I got a lot of stares. When we stopped our car at a light, I could often feel the eyes of the driver next to us, could hear them thinking, "Man, that's one awful-looking kid! Where are her eyebrows?" Occasionally I'd freak them out by pulling off my prosthetic leg and holding it up next to my face. One time, I saw a cop staring at me from the next car over. I looked him right in the eye and slowly lifted the wig off my head. His mouth shot open and his eyes bugged out. I guess I didn't lose *all* of my sense of humor.

Just before I'd gotten sick, we'd finally moved out of my

grandparents' house and into our own little apartment in a low-income housing neighborhood not far away. The day I left the hospital, my mom parked in front of our building in a handicapped spot and helped me out of the backseat. She hefted me into her arms and carried me up three flights. Our apartment door looked so normal to me—no hospital logo, no name labels, no smell of disinfectant masking sickness, just an ordinary, scratched-up wooden door. It was beautiful. And an even more beautiful sight greeted me behind it: Rugs and furniture that didn't need to be wiped down with antibacterial spray every day. Our school art on the fridge.

"Mom!" I said, first thing. "My Atari!" I had my priorities.

I pushed my crutches under my arms and hobbled over to the room I shared with my sister, Loren. I sighed. Rainbow bedspread, rainbow rug, rainbow poster. Awesome. Kermit the Frog, Miss Piggy. Muppet after Muppet via poster and stuffed toy. There was my 45 player with its little stack of records. There were my sister's Scott Baio posters—I'd even missed those, though I had no idea what she saw in him. But then my eyes traveled to my softball and gymnastics trophies, reminders of an active life I'd never get back. I looked away and moved to the bunk bed, threw my crutches aside and lay facedown on the bottom mattress. The bedspread smelled good, like home. But home was full of the old me, the dancer and athlete me, the normal girl with two legs.

One night, my mom helped me get dressed up, and we headed out to the Kosair Charities building in downtown Louisville. It was time to thank the group that had saved us from financial ruin.

The Cat and the Cripple

Our insurance policy covered eighty percent of the hospital costs. But when you're in a cancer ward for two years, the remaining twenty percent becomes an overwhelming sum. My mother simply couldn't pay, and determined she'd have to file for bankruptcy. Before finishing the forms, though, she reached out to the Shriners, who were affiliated with the hospital charities. They paid off our debt entirely.

So that night, we stood before a room full of seniors, many sporting the classic Shriner fez, and talked about what the group had done for me and my family. As grateful as I was, it was a hard night. I was a kid surrounded by hundreds of older people who wanted to hold my hand and tell me how sorry they were for me. Then it was home to bed, exhausted, to turn out the light and look forward to another day of chemo.

The only thing that I thought could help me feel better would be finally having the pet I'd dreamed of, a neutral and loyal friend. Maybe a kitten! (Now I'd say "companion animal," but back then, like everyone else, I called cats and dogs "pets.") When we'd lived at my grandparents' house, I wasn't allowed to have one, but now that we were in a place of our own, why not?

"I don't know, Jenny," my mom said when I started my begging campaign. "I don't think it's a good idea. Animals carry lots of germs. You know what the doctors are saying. . . ."

I can't blame my mother for being hesitant. Chemo wreaks havoc with the immune system, much like AIDS does. I easily caught colds, I developed frequent bladder infections, and my hands often sprouted painfully embarrassing warts. When I went out in public, I sometimes had to wear a surgical mask over my nose and mouth so I wouldn't catch anything. I knew how compromised I was. My doctors wouldn't even allow me to have my ears pierced—something I wanted desperately so that people wouldn't mistake me for a boy with my bald head and flat chest. (After a lot of begging, Dr. Patel relented on that, but he insisted on doing it himself in a sterile environment with a syringe needle . . . and boy did that hurt. I still have lopsided holes because of his unskilled (and painful!) piercing technique, but hey, I got to wear earrings.

Yet when it came to a pet, my obsession and *need* for one outweighed the risk of a cat-scratch infection. Finally, Mom and I asked Dr. Patel.

"Her white cell count's been good lately, Judy," he said. "With as much time as she's having to spend at home, I'd say the benefits outweigh the risks." Not a day after that conversation, Mom took Loren and me to her coworker's house, where a litter of kittens had been born a few weeks before.

When I sat down with those kittens, it took about ten seconds to notice the runt: underweight, outnumbered, a little scared. When she toddled over to me on dime-size paws, that was that.

My mother looked worried. "I think there might be something wrong with her," she said. She cocked her head and narrowed her eyes at the kitten.

I looked at Mom and said, "Well, there's something wrong with me, but that's okay, right?"

Her mouth tightened, and then her shoulders relaxed and she nodded. I was pretty good at guilt by then. But I also felt compelled to adopt the kitten who was most in need of special attention. Seeing a little somebody who stood out awkwardly, who might have been picked on or pushed away, brought out my empathy.

I held the scared little kitty on my lap in the backseat on the way home, Loren next to me, cooing at her. I put my hand on her back. She was smaller than our backyard squirrels and so delicate that I worried I could break her in half. "Do we have anything for her to eat?" I asked. I rummaged through the wrappers in a Burger King bag at my feet and fed her a cold french fry.

By the time we got home, I was pooped. The trip was much longer than my frequent hospital runs, and those were pretty much my only outings at that time. Loren went to the sofa and picked up a book, and I retreated to our room, crawling into bed. I perched my new little friend on my chest, thinking that, for a baby, this must be an exhausting adventure. After about five seconds, she started batting at wrinkles in the rainbow bedspread. Then she jumped down to the floor and began to explore her new digs. Soon she started attacking imaginary things on our moss-green shag carpet, like a lioness on a hunt. She zipped and zagged across the floor, stopping on occasion to ready a pounce, butt wiggling to and fro, and then she'd be off again. She was so much fun to watch, but what I wanted more than anything was for her to crawl up on my lap so I could cuddle her.

Little kids can be pretty gross. For me, this mostly manifested in a fascination with bodily fluids and yucky bio-matter in general. (I've hung on to that fascination to this day, which makes lancing pig abscesses easier for me than it might be for others.) Boogers were a big hit with me, and I named my new friend just that: Booger. "Could we at least call her 'Boogie'?" my mom begged. And Boogie stuck, a shortened version that could pass for charming.

The Lucky Ones

Later that night, as Boogie ran around my room at what seemed like a hundred miles per hour, I could only lie there. It was strange to be around so much energy when I had so little. Still, I wanted to bond and play with her. I reached over to pick up a notebook by the bed, tore the corner off a page, and rolled it into a tight ball. She followed my movements, spellbound by the crinkling sound. I tossed the ball across the floor and she pounced. Her fuzzy paw was hardly bigger than the wad, and she reached out to grab it, pushing it farther away in the process. Then she leapt on it and flipped onto her back. I laughed. She looked like a tiny otter holding a clam to her chest.

I made a shadow puppet on the wall, and she stared at it, rapt. I wiggled my fingers, and she pounced with a clunk at the wall. I envied her energy, and I envied her lack of awareness about the realities of life. "So this is home, Boogie," I told her. "I hope you'll be happy here. We'll play Boogie-is-a-lioness all you want."

I didn't realize that animals were really capable of complex emotions until I got to know Boogie. She could be even moodier than I was—which I didn't think was possible. I could soon tell when she was cranky or lonely or happy or just wanted to be left in peace. I talked to her the way I talked to a friend. When I would cry, she would often come over to investigate, batting at my mouth to stop my wailing or comforting me by licking the tears off my cheek—something she continued to do throughout our life together.

The closer Boogie and I became, the less time I spent thinking about my victimhood; now I began to think of hers. What must it have been like for her to be pulled away from her mother and siblings, carried away by strangers from the only home she'd known, and driven off to a random house with a random child? Where did people get the right to do that? Others had made choices for both of us, determining our fates, our lives. Animals, like kids, don't have equality when it comes to matters of importance. Why did some seemingly random men in white coats have the right to say it was okay to have my leg cut off?

I felt compelled to give Boogie the best life I possibly could, in order to right the wrong of her being taken away from her family. That feeling of responsibility for Boogie and an awareness about companion animals' vulnerability in general stayed with me all of her eighteen years. And it positioned me to consider the quality of life of billions of other creatures living and dying alongside us.

....

2

The Flying Leg

ecan was a young hen when she came to Woodstock Farm
Animal Sanctuary (WFAS). A kind woman who was pet-sitting
for people she hardly knew found Pecan cowering in the corner of
a shed where she, along with several dozen other hens, was being
kept for her eggs. It was no factory-farm operation, but there were
many signs that the chickens were not well cared for. When Pecan
arrived, I could definitely see why she'd be noticeable in a crowd of
birds: Her left foot was twisted, curled unnaturally up on itself,
and she could barely walk. It was unbearable to see her struggle to
stand, one leg extended awkwardly forward with the foot turned
inward. She would balance herself on her good leg and then try to
shift her weight to the curled-in foot, only to slide forward—almost
into a split—and lose her balance, extending her wings to try to
steady herself. I was determined to find a way to fix the problem.
Nothing like an I-can't-walk story to get me going.

I did some research for answers and found one: curly toe syndrome, caused by a riboflavin deficiency early in life. I was appalled,

yet happy to find that curly toe is completely curable. A standard farm would not consider it worth the trouble of correcting, and the bird would probably die, unable to reach food and water or have reasonable mobility among the crowd of other birds. Why wouldn't the farm fix it? Well, I could hop online right now, pull out my credit card, buy twenty-five laying chicks for $37.25, and have them shipped on over. Yes, you heard that right: the standard way egg operations—large *and* small—get their chicks is from a hatchery through the mail, like a new cell phone or DVD. Shipping regulations say nothing about food, water, weather—as long as the birds are delivered, alive or dead, within seventy-two hours, no problem. Millions of chicks are delivered dead each year. For hatcheries and farms, that's just an acceptable economic loss. (Places like McMurray Hatchery in Iowa ship an average of 100,000 chicks every week to buyers.) But hey, you get a discount for buying in bulk, so no need to worry if a few aren't "viable," right? In fact, if you look at the shipping policies of these hatcheries, they'll instruct you not to "count the dead ones," since they don't expect them all to make it and will ship extras to compensate.

With that attitude toward birds, why should a farmer care about a crippled foot? Let her die—replacements are a phone call away.

Well, that's obviously not our philosophy. I gathered Pecan onto my lap as I read more about curly toe. Once she settled, she began to relax, and I gently massaged her little foot and stretched it out flat against my palm. "All right, little lady," I said. "Let's see what we can do for you."

Once I knew enough about the syndrome, I called a vet to see if it was possible to correct it in a bird Pecan's age. Though vets are by no means accustomed to caring for animals who are usually culled rather than cured, this one ventured that he thought the leg could indeed be straightened and that he had seen it work for exotic birds.

The next day I started Pecan on an oral B complex (riboflavin is a B vitamin) to correct her deficiency. Then I accessed my inner MacGyver and got to work on a splint. I bent a tongue depressor until it partially snapped into an L shape. Next, I stretched and spread out Pecan's curled toes and taped them to a piece of plastic mesh so her foot wouldn't curl. I had all the makings of a brace to keep her foot flat and her leg straight.

I also fashioned a supporting sling out of a canvas grocery bag, cutting holes for her legs, a slit down the front for her neck and head, and a poop chute for necessary chicken business. Now that she was taped and slung, I started walking her, slowly, on my living room carpet, Doug holding the sling, me down on the floor moving Pecan's feet for her. We must have looked crazy. But wouldn't any dog or cat lover do the same? We worked on Pecan about twenty minutes at a time, three or four times a day, holding both of her feet at the proper angle. I was doing most of the work, but the idea was to remind her of what normal walking was like. She seemed to get used to this within days, and I started seeing results within a week. The grapes and applesauce she got as rewards for physical therapy didn't hurt any. Who doesn't like treats?

Two weeks in, Pecan was able to walk on her own. One afternoon I gently removed her sling for the final test. I set her down on the carpet, and Doug and I watched her tentatively bear weight on the foot, then walk, wings flapping madly, from the sofa to the coffee table and past the dog bed, all on her own. We helped the process by enticing her with the coveted grapes. I cheered her on with frantic clapping.

Within a month of starting treatment, Pecan was running around with the other hens. As she acclimated to walking and running, she'd use her wings to steady herself. But pretty soon she looked just like her twenty-four fellow flock members, and Doug and I couldn't get enough of watching her scratch and stretch and roam around her yard. She even mastered a sexy little strut around our first rescued rooster, Rio. Ridiculous smiles on our faces, we stood there and stared, turning only to high-five, never more proud.

Pecan was an extremely affectionate bird. As much as she loved her new flock, she'd always come running back to our house whenever she heard our front door swing open—on the lookout for treats and people-company. If people could see amazing personalities like Pecan's for themselves, maybe chicken patties and Buffalo wings, composed of slaughtered egg-laying hens, would be less popular. . . .

■ ■ ■ ■

By seventh grade, I was up to a healthy weight; my hair, eyebrows, and eyelashes were finally starting to grow in; and I was gaining energy by the day. I had undergone nearly two awful years of chemo post amputation, and the regime of toxic drugs was finally over. Though it would be another three years of regular bone scans before doctors could confirm that all traces of cancer were gone, I was sure I had beat the disease and was ready to get on with life. Gradually, I started to do that. There were interruptions in this flow, though, as I tried to acclimate to new and better models of artificial limbs. I started with some real clunkers—ranging from stark metal rods to the I-stole-it-from-a-mannequin look—and as my wound healed and I grew, I had to make adjustments and try new models, a tiresome and often painful exercise.

Finally I met Don, the brains behind my first "good" leg. Don was an ex-firefighter. "I lost a foot on the job," he told me, treating me like a person, not a fake leg or a kid. "Nobody knew how to make me a good prosthetic, so I thought, hey, let me try, and I went back to school." He'd been where I was, and it felt good to know that he genuinely understood. Sure enough, the new leg was more comfortable, and it was also more realistic (though not to say actually realistic) than previous ones. It even had "toenails," and after my final fitting, Don handed me a bag. "Here you go, sweetie," he said. "Hope you like the color." Inside was a bottle of pink nail polish.

I became so comfortable in my new leg that soon after I received it, I was able to walk with a normal gait and skip and jog a little bit if I really needed to. I even began doing cartwheels again. Inspired by my renewed athletic ability, I decided to go along with some girlfriends and try out for a community league's cheerleading team. Making the squad was a huge boost to my self-esteem, and my buddies Cindy and Rachel made it, too, sweetening the triumph. We'd go to the squad leader's house and practice our half-time dance routine to "Eye of the Tiger." (We idolized her—she was a *college* cheerleader.) Then we'd pile into a pyramid. The fake leg would sometimes dig into the other cheerleaders' backs, so I was often on the bottom.

With my new fancy leg, I was feeling better, more confident than

I had in a long time. As I cheered the home team, the Nuggets, at those basketball games, I felt downright *normal*, except for my super-short hair, which couldn't be helped, since it was just growing back. Leg warmers were fortunately very much in style, and my cream-colored pair covered in multicolored balls masked the fake leg that lurked below my uniform skirt. And luckily, I still had my knee, which meant a range of motion enough to kick and flip and be cute and enthused like any good cheerleader.

Then came that heated tournament game. As I cheered my heart out before the packed stands, I felt confident enough to try a cartwheel/round-off combo. These were old hat to me from my gymnastics days, and I'd been practicing on our lawn for weeks, so there was no reason to hold back. When the team scored at a crucial point of the game, I looked at the throng of fans on their feet and declared it time for the show-off moves. I lunged onto my hands and flung my feet into the air to perform the combo. That's when it happened: My leg detached, spectacularly. Think of that pivotal moment in *2001: A Space Odyssey*, when the bone flies through the air, only more dramatic. It shot off, spinning toes over calf through the air into the middle of the court, and finally landed with a loud, inelegant *CLUNK* between two bewildered players. They both looked down at it, silent and agape, then looked at each other. Their coach hadn't trained them for *this*.

From there, everything happened in slow motion: Hundreds of mouths falling open, plenty of gasps, and then a deadly silence; a mother reaching to cover her son's eyes; my own mother standing up to call to my best friend, "CINDY! GET THE LEG!" Cindy just stared at her, frozen. I went numb. Then my brain snapped on long enough to tell me to burst into tears and hop, then scooch on my butt, face glowing red, toward the gym door. It was the longest dozen yards I'd ever traveled, especially by butt. I wanted to get as far from that place as I could and never go back. I crawled into the girls' bathroom, locked myself into a stall, bawling, and waited for my mother to grab the leg and come find me. In the safety of that bathroom, I recalled, sobbing, the shocked expressions of the couple of boys on the team whom I had crushes on. How could I face my fellow cheerleaders or any fan or player again? So much for my plan to pass for "normal."

I've long since figured out that humor is my friend, that it puts people at ease and situations into perspective. So I love telling this wacky story, acting it out. I pantomime the mother covering her son's eyes in slow motion at the horror of the leg shooting through the air like a cannonball. I impersonate my stricken mother shouting at half speed, *"CINNNNNNDYYYYY! GEEEEET THE LEEEEEGGGGG!!"* I describe the team stopping mid-play to watch the beet-red, one-legged cheerleader flee via her ass.

But kids can bounce back amazingly well. Turned out that I *was* able to face my fellow cheerleaders again and laugh about it with them. No matter the setbacks, I spent more and more time reconnecting with friends and getting the hang of school. By ninth grade, nausea, pain, and fatigue distant memories and my leg solid under me, I started feeling and acting like a regular teenager.

I was from the south side of Louisville, so being a regular teenager meant cruising up and down the same strip of Dixie Highway in beat-up cars, peach wine coolers in hand, blasting Ratt or some other heavy metal band and singing along to every last lyric. I'd tease my partially bleached hair tall in our cramped bathroom, and then a boyfriend would pick me up, his mullet equally groomed, and we'd roll out of the housing complex past tanning salons, car washes, and pawn shops. We'd meet up with friends and other raucous teens in the Hardee's parking lot, eat burgers and fries, smoke cigarettes, and hang out in the glow of undercarriage neon from the boys' Trans Ams. I became the definition of a rebellious youth.

To keep myself in Virginia Slim menthols and to start saving for a car of my own someday, I got a job just where you'd expect an animal lover to work: McDonald's.

I might have been grossed out by the greasy, pimply guys who worked the grill, but I ate what they fried. I'd watch the perfect frozen circles brown on the grill and make no connection to animals at all. The atmosphere was sterile and push-button, alien to anything alive—animal or, for that matter, vegetable. It was the opposite of a homey kitchen, a warm, bountiful, nourishing place, and it was easy for me to feel I was entering some sort of automated zone divorced from the real world.

I went home to Boogie each night and didn't think it strange to cuddle one furry animal and watch another one sizzle. I had no idea that McDonald's is the world's largest purchaser of beef, that it builds its Big Macs by buying from enormous plants that process 800,000 pounds of hamburger a day from thousands of cows at a time. I didn't know that many of those are dairy cows too old and wasted to produce enough milk to justify keeping them alive, so they become cheap hamburger at four or five years of age (when a healthy cow could easily live to be twenty). I had no idea that for its

McChicken sandwich, McDonald's uses "electrical immobilization" to kill chickens, which means hanging them upside down in metal shackles, causing terrible bruises, hemorrhages, and broken bones. I didn't know the kill line goes so fast that the birds' throats are often not fully slit before they're plunged into tanks of scalding-hot water to loosen their feathers. I had no idea that McDonald's suppliers, such as agricultural giant Cargill, are responsible for a huge amount of Amazonian deforestation for soy crops to feed animals, and that sixty-five to seventy percent of Brazilian rainforest has been clear-cut for cattle grazing. No, I didn't know any of that— plus, I was saving up for a car.

Meanwhile, I'm not sure I even knew what a vegetarian was. I was almost out of high school when I met my first one, and she didn't exactly make me want to join her. She was a punk rocker, and while that may have been cool in other parts of the country, where we were, it was just plain weird. We shook our heads at her combat boots, Day-Glo hair, and "Meat Is Murder" T-shirt. The way she ate was just part of her kookiness to us, a way to get attention and at the same time stand apart. I remember asking her why she was a vegetarian, but nothing she said kept me from walking back over to the acid-washed side of the school cafeteria and enjoying a slice of pepperoni pizza with my pals.

When I wasn't working, going out with boys, or fighting with my mom, I was doing what Southside girls did: fight each other. That's just the way things got settled in my (red)neck of the woods. I wonder if all the meat we ate played a role in our aggression; after all, my two biggest knock-down drag-outs were in a Hardee's parking lot and on a McDonald's counter, respectively.

The Lucky Ones

....

We were still inside the Hardee's that first time when my friend and a girl from rival Valley High started trash-talking each other over a guy they both had dated. We were just leaving when I heard one of her friends yell, "Go get her, Rhonda! I'll take her peg-leg friend." I could feel my nostrils and my temper flare. Unfortunately, mean nicknames were part of life from the time I started back to school. The kids loved "Peg Leg," but "Long John Silver" and just plain "Gimpy" for the less imaginative were other favorites. When I got frustrated enough about it, I tended to use my fists.

"How dare you—you don't know me! I'll kick your [expletive] ass!" I yelled back. Before I could even ask my friend to hold my earrings, the girl kicked my fake leg out from under me—on purpose. I thunked right over. I could hear my head crack on the pavement. As she pounded my face, all I could focus on was maneuvering my leg back on, which I finally did. Needless to say I lost that fight, but having my leg come off in public or even bringing attention to it in any way was beyond humiliating. I tried my best to hide it however I could for years to come, even though everyone knew.

Then there was the McDonald's fight, which cost me my job—but on the other hand, that's a good thing. I remember being upset because my supervisor, at the last minute, told me to sweep and mop the lobby before I left, and that would make me late for my date that night. Amy, a coworker whom I didn't always mesh with, started mocking me when I complained.

"Oh, well then, let's roll out the red carpet for Miss Jenny Brown," she sneered, trying to get a rise out of me. "Hey, we'll just do all the work so poor Jenny can get out of here." My teeth clenched and my nostrils did their thing again. We ended up literally rolling over and over on the gray countertop. Eventually she hauled me over to the drive-thru window and hung my head out of it with her hands around my throat. That's when I punched her in the face. And got fired.

Am I proud to say I won as many fights as I lost? It's a pretty shameful memory, but it's how things were done in my neighborhood and at that age. Cruise and flirt, eat burgers, smoke cigarettes, listen to Duran Duran (I had other tastes besides heavy metal, of course) while lying in the tanning bed or in the sun wearing Crisco, and pummel each other when "necessary." It took me a long time to question any of those behaviors. And to this day, if a visitor wisecracks about a pig looking tasty, my inner Louisville knows there's a quick and satisfying solution. Fortunately, my outer Woodstock usually prevails. Usually.

3

Taking the Red Pill

S ome animals arrive at the sanctuary terrified, fearful of every-one around them. Sometimes they're like Jack, a goat who was seized from a storefront slaughterhouse (or "live-kill" market). He was being kept for breeding in the same room where other animals were strung up by their hind legs and had their throats slit, day after day. He arrived at WFAS so scared that at first he tried to ram us against a barn wall. Or like Cora, a hen who had escaped from another live-kill market in the city, featherless, debeaked, and only just released from a tiny cage crammed with other laying hens; we thought she might have a heart attack the first time we handled her. These poor creatures have endured such anxiety and fear that they can't imagine kindness or a show of concern for their well-being. After the abuse of standard farming practices, they assume that this place, too, will be a scary one.

Not true of Patsy and Judy.

Patsy and Judy were the first piglets to join our older, estab-lished pig herd, and we had no idea how their introduction would go. Their previous home was in rural Maryland, where they were being kept with no shelter by a man who'd been forbidden to own animals because of a record of abuse. This man, no surprise, kept on raising animals anyway for fast cash at livestock auctions. He thought if he kept them deep in the woods, no one would find them. Fortunately, he was wrong. A hiker came across their secluded pen and contacted local animal control. The officers discovered his emaciated horses tangled in their tethers, along with a poorly kept litter of piglets, their mother already gone. There was no food or water anywhere in sight.

A lot of the discussions about animal welfare and rights these days focus on factory farms, and for good reason—the overwhelming majority of farm animals live in that particular brand of misery. But we who rescue animals see and hear of case after case of "local" and "small" farmers abusing, neglecting, or abandoning their animals, too.

The officers down in Maryland immediately confiscated the horses and piglets and called Farm Sanctuary, the first U.S. haven for farm animals. I'd actually trained at Farm Sanctuary in upstate New York for close to a year before starting my own sanctuary, and the staff there knew that Woodstock Farm Animal Sanctuary might have room for pigs.

The shelter director at Farm Sanctuary, Susie Coston, my old mentor and one of my dearest friends and comrades to this day, called me to see if we had room for any of the survivors. We were more than happy to help. Soon two rambunctious piglets arrived, eager to check out their new home, each already weighing close to fifty pounds. I named them Patsy Ruth and Judy Lynn after my mom and grandmother. They both reacted well to the news and still love to tell their friends that there are fat, happy pigs named after them at their (grand)daughter's animal sanctuary.

The young girls hadn't been socialized with humans much, but within hours of their arrival, they were flopping over on their sides for belly rubs. A very good sign. We put them in an isolation pen inside the pig barn, where they could be fully vetted and kept separate until the other pigs got used to their presence. Several of the older pigs came right over to check out the newcomers. They could get nose to nose with them through the slatted pen wall. The older sows were the first to come over, vocalizing gently while trying to practically inhale the piglets. They were so interested in the new arrivals, and the newbies were excited to meet them in a way I hadn't imagined, especially considering that they probably hadn't met other pigs outside their siblings and mother. Then Stubby, our biggest male by far, came over. First, he nosed and talked to the older sows. Then he turned toward the piglets and engaged in the same soft, openmouthed grunts. Wilbur joined in, then Cromwell, and before we knew it, all the pigs were lining up and crowding around to meet the new girls. Everything was going swimmingly until grumpy Oliver, an older pig with a temper, tried to push big Stubby out of the way. Both started to growl and scream and hurl their giant heads at each other, which is the sometimes scary and incredibly loud way adult pigs tend to work things out. This terrified the girls, who ran to the other side of their pen, squealing in fear, and I, of course, stood by to comfort them. Luckily, spats like that blow over quickly with the pigs. Ten minutes later Stubby and Oliver were side by side in their straw beds, buddies again.

After a week in their own pen and outdoor yard, under our

watchful eyes, we introduced the girls to the rest of the herd. Patsy and Judy were brave around the older pigs but had to learn when to leave adults alone. They could move a lot quicker than the senior pigs, so they always escaped without injury when they got a little too rambunctious with their elders. Soon they became comfortable and intuitive about their place in the herd. They had ravenous appetites and at feeding time would squeal at the top of their lungs until the gate opened, allowing them access to the troughs. And boy, did they grow—even on their low-fat diets of produce, horse pellets (most pig feed has animal by-products added, including porcine blood!), and their absolute favorite, the occasional bagel or partial loaf of bread. Their days were spent out in the pasture, rooting in the ground side by side, mixed with occasional playful dashes across the field, chasing each other. On warm days, they would pass out in their muddy pig pond when they grew tired. They were and still are as close as two sisters can be, which is to say they can be mean and grumpy to each other and then best friends minutes later. When they sleep for the night inside the pig barn, we always see them spooned together in a pile of sweet-smelling rye straw that they have meticulously worked into a suitably comfortable bed. As for people, those two come right up to us for a scratch, which *always* leads to them flopping over for a belly rub. They absolutely love belly rubs. When they were tiny, you could rub each tummy by making tiny circles with the palm of your hand. But as they grew into six-hundred-pound adults, it started to take a lot more energy to do it. Now it's like washing a car in *Karate Kid*—wax on, wax off. It takes some pretty broad strokes to cover the span of their massive bellies, but it's their ultimate bliss, and naturally we aim to please!

After the pig barn is cleaned, I love to open the bales of straw to lay on the ground for comfort. Word must spread that it's happening because many of the pigs come in to help with this favorite task. Patsy is especially keen on this, and gets very excited when she sees the bales come in. She can't even wait until I remove the string from the straw bale before she grabs a big mouthful and starts to make a bed for herself. Next she'll scurry around, evenly distributing piles on the barn floor for everybody else. If a few pigs are already napping, she and others will shake mouthfuls over them until they are covered with a cozy straw blanket. It's like watching a nine-hundred-pound bird build a nest.

■ ■ ■ ■

It's safe to say that many Americans will go through their entire lives never even seeing a pig in person, let alone watching one with a name build a nest. And since they're not "cuddly" or constantly seeking human attention or affection (well, some do), they're easy to disconnect from. Author Michael Pollan put it well: "There's a schizoid quality to our relationship with animals, in which sentiment and brutality exist side by side. Half the dogs in America will receive Christmas presents this year, yet few of us pause to consider the miserable life of the pig—an animal easily as intelligent as a dog—that becomes the Christmas ham."

Pigs are the fourth-most intelligent animal on the planet; only apes, dolphins, and elephants are smarter. So Pollan was wrong about one thing: Pigs are more intelligent than dogs—and, in fact, most three-year-old children. I'm sure even the many people who

have studied pig intelligence have been surprised by their findings, given our cultural construct that pigs are simply where bacon
and pork chops come from. In fact it's trendy these days for hipsters to wear clothes that say things like "I Love Bacon" or "Bacon
Makes Everything Better!" It makes me sad how so far removed
people are from the reality that bacon came from a sentient animal who lived a life of deprivation, pain, frustration, and fear, all
for food that we have no nutritional need for.

Researchers, most notably Dr. Stanley Curtis, who was an inter-
nationally renowned professor at the University of Illinois and
Penn State, have long studied pigs' remarkable intelligence. Pigs
can learn words and phrases easily and remember them for years,
and they are perfectly capable of abstract thinking. They can find
their way home from a great distance, and looking at computer
screens, they can distinguish between squiggle patterns they've
seen and ones they haven't. They can be taught to play video games.
They dream. Their complex social dynamics rival primates'. Pig
mamas actually "sing" to their young while nursing, teaching them
to recognize the vocalizations of their own mothers. These are just
some examples of the sophistication of pigs' brains, and we live
with the evidence every day at the sanctuary (though, no, our pigs
do not have PlayStation).

But amazing as these facts are, I wonder, should they even matter? Must animals be intelligent for humans to have compassion
and empathy toward them? To be spared misery? We don't make
those distinctions for humans in the United States; there's no IQ
qualifier in the Constitution. Abusers can't get off the hook with,

"But, Officer, he's just dumb." That would be an injustice and an infringement of our rights. Ahh, but we're talking about animals who *don't* have rights—who live within a human-designed system of privileges that don't extend to them. As the nineteenth-century philosopher and animal rights activist Jeremy Bentham said, "The question is not, can they reason? Nor, can they talk? But, can they suffer?" I'd like us to be compassionate, not because tests show similarities between our intelligence and theirs, but because imposing pain, fear, loneliness, and imprisonment on sentient beings of any intelligence simply isn't right.

There wasn't a question about where I was going to go to college. Money talks, but so does the lack of it: It was going to be the University of Louisville for me. But as close as U of L was to where I grew up, nothing was the same—except maybe the Southern drawls. I walked among the lush lawns, tall white columns, and clock towers with a bit of wide-eyed wonder. The other students were my introduction to Louisville's diversity. There were kids from the east side of town who wore argyle and talked about private school and European ski trips. There were downtown kids who wore Goth clothes and spiky armbands and went to punk shows. There were west-side kids, mostly black, who wore baggy clothes and gold chains and played Run-DMC. Only then did I make my first Jewish friend, my first lesbian friend, my first atheist friend. I met people from other states and other countries. Someone told me about the L.L.Bean catalog; someone else showed me her tongue piercing. Both of those items sort of blew my mind. I still bought my clothes at a discount store called Fashion Shop and had only recently quit wearing my hair as big as it could get. Interacting with these people, some of whom grew up a neighborhood away and some whose native countries I'd have trouble finding on a map, caused some internal shifts in me.

During college orientation week, I wandered into the student union lobby and browsed a line of information tables, picking up interesting handouts. Before long I found myself in front of a pile of pamphlets from PETA (People for the Ethical Treatment of Animals). The animal photos on their covers caught my attention. I picked up one about the circus and one about animal experimentation and went off to the student lounge.

On a giant orange sectional couch, I read pamphlets that turned my brain and my heart upside down. Turns out the circus was no circus. All those years of exciting Ringling Bros. shows I'd loved were actually, I was seeing, the story of baby elephants torn from their families to lead long, miserable, lonely lives. I had been clapping and cheering for that? Then I read about animal experimentation, and it brought an even more personal chill: Had I been cured of disease only by the grace of countless miserable lives and ugly deaths? And what of the less "noble" causes? What about animal misery for the sake of mascara?

I sat in the lounge watching students absorbed in conversation, sipping soda, laughing. Someone asked me where the registration office was, snapping me out of my reverie. Things looked the same, but they weren't for me. This world I hadn't thought much about was dreadful, but it was reality, and the genie wouldn't stuff back in the bottle.

I set down the pamphlets and rummaged through my backpack for the course catalog. I cracked it open with an eye to seeing which classes might provide avenues to explore these issues; maybe if I learned more, if I could focus what was swirling through my head, I'd feel less overwhelmed. There were no animal rights or humane education courses back then and no animal ethics and theory to be had. But one class jumped out at me: public speaking. I read in its description that the course required students to choose a semester-long topic—that meant I could focus on animal issues and get credit. I signed right up.

My first speech for the class was about laboratory animals. Through those endless chemo treatments, I'd never once thought about what cats, dogs, rabbits, mice, and primates went through so the drugs could make their way to me. I might have hated that chemo, but I'm sure they hated it a lot more—and at least I was getting it to save my life, not to sacrifice it. I started to wonder about how many animals had been tortured—and "torture" is the accurate term—so that, for instance, the researchers could determine lethal doses of the drugs I was given as chemotherapy.

I was wading into complicated waters here. Some of the articles I read argued that saving human lives was worth taking the lives of other species, but other research told me it was rarely that simple. Even animals used to supposedly save human lives are often dying in vain. Animal studies for cancer are notoriously unreliable. Animal bodies are different enough from ours that most tests are useless or worse. When doctors Jean and Ray Greek studied animal testing, they found that different drugs have drastically different effects, depending on species and even genders. As Ray put it, if we can't tell how a drug will react in a female as opposed to male human, "What, pray tell, makes us think that a mouse is going to predict what that drug is going to do?" He goes on to declare, "This cross-species testing concept has outlived its usefulness by about a century."

In fact, I began to understand that animal testing actually *costs* human lives. Plenty of drugs that passed muster with animals have shown to be harmful and even lethal for humans.

If someone had sat me down the week before I started working on my speech class project and asked, "Why do we test on animals?" I would have told them, "Well, it's so that humans can survive." I wasn't aware of the issue's complexities, nor had I ever seen the injustice in imposing such experiments on animals for our own gain. But what I was even more ignorant about—and what isn't complex at all—was methodical animal abuse for the sake of makeup or hair dye. Since my friends and I were single-handedly keeping Clairol, Maybelline, and Alberto V05 in business, I felt pretty shameful about that. And Aqua Net? Please—I had put those people's kids through college. But before it got to my bathroom cabinet, that hairspray was used as a torture device: Jeez, I wonder what would happen to a rabbit who had hairspray repeatedly directed into her eyes, only her head sticking out of a locked box? Let's perform a scientific experiment and find out. Disgusting.

I read that not only are these tests conducted for "new" products that are pretty much identical to their old counterparts, but they are repeated over and over, partly because of outdated mandates and partly because of the lack of a nationwide database that shares information about previous testing results. There must be great job security in the field of laboratory research.

Taking the Red Pill

I came to understand that cosmetics aren't required to be tested on animals, but in our litigious society, many large companies do it Just In Case. Just in case someone smears their eyeballs with hand lotion every day for a month? Just in case someone eats ten sticks of deodorant? "Look, the fact is that the overwhelming majority of animal testing doesn't even pay lip service to saving human lives," I told my classmates during my presentation. "Its job is to make sure mouthwash and eye shadow companies don't get sued. Is that ethical?"

Mercifully, some companies don't test at all; they rely on natural or pretested ingredients. Even for new ingredients, there are so many effective alternatives to these tests that there's just no need to cause profound misery to living beings. For instance, pharmaceutical tests can often be efficiently and accurately performed using donated human blood. And other drugs and products can be tested "in silico" instead of "in vitro," meaning through computer simulation rather than by using living beings. From heart disease to drug toxicity to asthma, computers have been shown to test successfully minus the cruelty. L'Oréal now tests skin care products using human skin cell cultures, having changed its policy in response to consumer demand. This choice is cost-effective and even more accurate, since it utilizes our own species' skin and can even adjust for skin tone and aging.

And yet major companies like Colgate-Palmolive, Johnson & Johnson, and Procter & Gamble continue to use outdated, cruel tests. I researched, for instance, the infamous Draize test, in which rabbits (chosen because their eyes can't tear up!) are forced to endure poison in their eyes day after day. I read about tests in which animals are strapped down, shaved, and slathered with skin "care" products to see how much would cause blistering and burning.

"Let's not forget about 'oral gavage,'" I told my class. "A tube is shoved down, say, a beagle puppy's throat and used to pump in household products, agrochemicals, and/or petrochemicals several times a day." I'd also read about chemicals injected into animals and chemical vapors that animals were forced to inhale. And primate tests that made the animals go crazy in their cages. And vivisection: Experimenting on conscious animals without sedation or pain meds in order to study their pain or the activity of their brains, or other horrible medical procedures. And of course, none of these animals had a life after their bodies had been used and used up: It was straight on the dead pile for all of them.

I realized that I needed to throw out every product in the house made by the aforementioned companies. Wow—that could have filled a shopping cart. Our toothpaste, shampoo, laundry detergent, and other products were all made by Procter & Gamble. Good-bye, Crest; good-bye, Neutrogena. We had Clorox, we had Arm & Hammer, we had Visine. My Hawaiian Tropic tanning lotion (hey, it was the '80s) had to go, and that gentle, pure Ivory (if the ads had any say in the matter) didn't deserve its reputation.

I cornered my mother and sister. "You can't believe how much blood is on our hands from having this stuff around!" I shouted. "Mom, don't buy Tide! Stop buying Lysol! We can live without these. Animals live terrified, miserable lives in laboratories and undergo horrendously cruel experiments."

"Let's just use what we have, Jenny," Mom would try to persuade me. "Plus, that other stuff is expensive, and I've got coupons for these."

"I'll buy it, then," I'd tell her. "I'll buy everything—you don't have to get it anymore."

I called and requested a dozen of PETA's cruelty-free wallet-size guides for my family and friends to carry around when we shopped. Eventually, all of us ended up liking the Good Stuff better anyway. We started using products from companies like Tom's of Maine, Jāsön, Nature's Gate, and Aubrey Organics. They smelled and worked just great, and once you've moved away from those harsh chemical-y smells and artificial colors, you're not eager to go back.

I may have been shattered by all of this new and chilling information, but my semester wasn't stopping there. My whole life I'd thought animals looked like they were having fun in the circus ring—it seemed like a symbiotic relationship between human and lion or elephant. Until I looked at that PETA leaflet in the student lounge, I had never thought about what these animals dealt with offstage, which was, of course, where almost all of their lives took place. I'd always loved seeing elephants, huge and majestic, at the zoo. Now I was reading about how deeply intelligent and emotional they were. I read about their enormous brains, similar to ours with respect to structure and sophistication. I read about their sense of humor, fierce maternal love, ability to mourn, appreciation for art and learning, and self-awareness. I read about their complex matriarch-led families: females and their offspring who are taught and nurtured by the older females; increasingly independent male groupings called "bull bands" that maintain a bond with the matriarchal relatives; and larger clans.

This was fascinating reading, but when I shut my books and looked up from my carrel in the library, I immediately pictured a lone, locked-up elephant at the Louisville Zoo. Here it came: the mixture of shame, sadness, and frustration that started to typify my mental state during every study session.

"Even we wily humans can't fly across the world, wrestle an adult male elephant, drag him back to America, and train him to balance a ball on his trunk," I explained to my classmates. "But we're wily enough to figure out another way—tear the babies from their moms and clans." Only the most vulnerable could be bullied into a life of captivity, misery, and servitude. And bullied they are: Elephants, along with their big cat and bear cousins, are routinely shocked, whipped, and beaten so that they'll perform "tricks" that make no sense to them. They are deprived of families, space, and play. As a result, of course, these animals are deeply distressed, physically and emotionally. I read that in the circus, there is no such thing as "positive reinforcement"—trainers use whips, electric prods, bullhooks, muzzles, and other torturous means. They break animals' spirits and their will through beatings.

And why? So someone can sit and watch an elephant step onto a box and stand on her hind legs? It seemed like such a throwback to disgraceful times in Western history when Africans were paraded before onlookers at world's fairs. Here was another kind of exploitation and oppression of one group to please another, so entrenched that most of us see it as nothing more than entertainment.

As soon as I'd written and delivered that speech, I had to turn my research attention to the next topic: farm animals. I crammed my brain full of information, determined to stare all this in the face, and all of it mortified me. But there were certain bits that stuck even more intensely than others. I kept thinking, for instance, about chickens on the slaughter line. They're shackled by the legs and moved along mechanically to slaughter, writhing, trying to right themselves, shitting on the workers. The workers slit their throats, but the line moves so quickly and the birds are so frantic that the workers can't kill all of them. Many birds are still alive when they arrive at the next part of the line: the vat of scalding water that loosens their feathers. Thousands of them are plunged in fully conscious. Thousands *every day*.

This would be bad enough, but at the same time I was researching slaughter practices, I was learning more about the animals themselves. The love of a mother hen for her chicks, the cleverness of pigs. So I was going back and forth between learning things that made me admire these species and things that were almost too appalling to think about. Egg-laying hens crammed so tight they can't lift their wings as their eggs drop and roll down to a conveyor belt. Mama pigs artificially inseminated and stuffed into crates until they give birth, only to have their babies pulled away to become Easter hams. The systematic, rampant, unnecessary cruelty to these very beings for the sake of Buffalo wings, cold cuts, and hot dogs.

And then there are the workers. Humans suffer in the slaughterhouse, too. Since few would choose to work in the hell of a slaughterhouse or feedlot, how do these industries fill positions? Not surprisingly, I read, by hiring the most vulnerable in our society: illegal immigrants, illiterate women, people of color in low-income communities, underage workers. Human Rights Watch, an international NGO dedicated to the protection and preservation of human rights, abhors factory-farm work, the most dangerous job in the

United States, and refers to it as rife with "systematic human rights abuses." HRW published an exhaustive study called "Blood, Sweat, and Fear" that blew the lid off the industry, citing "constant fear and risk," "severe, life-threatening, and sometimes life-ending injuries," and general "conditions, vulnerabilities, and abuses which violate human rights," including harassment of workers who try to claim workers' compensation for those severe injuries.

Reading about workers led me to another new and disturbing discovery: There are always those who, victimized themselves, lash out at those even more vulnerable and become oppressors. I saw undercover footage showing workers throwing chickens against a wall, punching and sitting on turkeys, beating and kicking pigs to death, dragging half-dead cows around by a leg with a chain and a tractor. I also read stories of workers sexually abusing animals. As if the day-to-day reality of life as a thinking, feeling commodity wasn't horrific enough.

This fits the sometime pattern of the abused becoming the abuser. Some workers, tired of being the low man on one or more totem poles in their own lives, lash out at beings even "lower" than they are. Other workers take out their frustration at the misery of their work on creatures who can't complain, retaliate, or get them in trouble, and their ears become deaf to the animals' screams. Other abusers are simply those with a penchant for violence who may be kept in check in other sectors of society but who have free rein in the hell of a slaughterhouse or farm.

Whatever abusers' reasons for perpetrating such sadistic crimes, the fact is that when people are allowed to hold power over vulnerable living beings, there are often horrifying results. Instead of getting counseling or support for suffering abuse or frustration themselves, these people are given knives and access to conscious, powerless beings.

My speeches were impassioned and earned me high marks, but the knowledge changed more than my transcript. I thought back on the Big Macs and McNuggets I'd sold and eaten, nothing more to me than a means to a paycheck. I decided right there at the U of L library that I'd have to make changes if I was going to live with myself. That was scary. I wanted to be a vegetarian, but my home and culture were entirely meat-centered—what would I eat? How would people see me? And another thing: I was trying to put all those years of ridicule I'd experienced since the amputation behind me—would this be a new topic for ridicule, and for feeling different?

I brought these questions home to my mom and sister. "I don't want to eat meat anymore," I told them. "I want to be a vegetarian. We love animals, so why do we eat them?"

My mom worried, like the rest of the world, "Where will you get your protein?!"

"Oh, Mom," I said. "That's brainwashing. Look, instead of a chicken burrito, you eat a bean burrito!"

"Is that all you're gonna eat?"

I thought of all the meals my mom made without meat. "Well, what about your gumbo? And I can have mushroom pizza instead of pepperoni. And what about fake-meat meatballs? I've heard about those."

Much to my relief, Mom and Loren were entirely supportive of my decision. They heard me out and couldn't help but agree. They, too, were big animal lovers, and besides a few worried questions about sufficient iron and such—questions I could easily answer, thanks to all those hours in the library—they decided to stand by me. We immediately agreed to remove beef and pork from our diets. I also stopped eating poultry right away, though Mom and Loren hung on to that for a while. We talked about what we'd replace those foods with. It was intimidating at first, but before long we found it wasn't as hard as we'd thought it would be. Instead of adding ground beef to the spaghetti sauce, we added TVP (texturized vegetable protein), which has the same texture and absorbs all the same flavors as ground beef. We made vegetable stew instead of beef stew. We moved the rice and beans to the center of the plate and dolled them up gloriously. It wasn't gourmet, but it was satisfying and filling and cheap, and just as important, we felt that we were Doing the Right Thing. Besides, when had food in my house ever been gourmet?

I started shopping at the only health food store in Louisville at the time, Rainbow Blossom, and got turned on to veggie burgers and tofu and all sorts of new, animal-free foods—and I loved it. A little while later, I stopped eating fish. They aren't sea vegetables, after all. They have nerve endings and feel pain, which is a great reason not to hurt them. But they also have intelligence, they utilize memory and cooperation, they recognize one another as individuals, they make decisions. Killing them unnecessarily for food (and killing outrageous numbers of their fellow fish and other marine life as ocean "bycatch" while fishing) struck me as wrong. And while aquaculture—raising fish in confinement—might do away with the bycatch issue, it is, in the words of Jonathan Safran Foer, "essentially underwater factory farming."

Chilling and life-changing as all this new knowledge was, I found it paradoxically freeing. For the first time, I was making decisions for myself about what I ate, what I chose to study, what I cared about. I wasn't doing what my mother or doctor or teacher told me to do. I was doing what my own value system was telling me to do: Learn, absorb, take action. And, in a further turn-around, I'd had my first experience of educating others. I was glad to know what I was part of, and I knew that some other people would be, too, so I brought my knowledge home and began getting to work influencing the people closest to me. My mother and sister began leaving meat off their plate (today they are mostly vegan), and my best friend since sixth grade, Tammy Pennington, was also inspired to go veg. She went on to marry my friend John Marcum, a match I made, and through the persuasive powers we females possess, he also became a vegetarian. They now have a teenage daughter, Olivia, who was raised vegetarian and proudly tells everyone that she thinks eating animals is wrong. Olivia has visited the sanctuary and says she'd like to start an animal sanctuary of her own someday. Be still, my beating heart! Olivia the goat got her name from my young friend.

During that time, I found myself looking at Boogie in a new way: She wasn't just an individual animal I cared about; she was a catalyst and my tie to the animal kingdom, a symbol of the closeness and respect I felt for the nonhumans in our midst. I bestowed more hugs and kisses on that kitty than she knew what to do with. During my research, I'd come across a quote from the writer Franz Kafka. He had become a vegetarian because of his empathy for animals, and one day while he was watching fish swim, he said, "Now at last I can look at you in peace; I don't eat you anymore."

Even though I'd obviously never envisioned ever eating Boogie or any domestic "pet," I felt a heightened sense of awareness and compassion toward all animals, and that changed the way I looked at her.

Still, Louisville was a lonely place to be a vegetarian back then. I knew only one other, my friend Julie, and she subsisted primarily on Taco Bell bean burritos. Home was a safe space where my mother chopped tofu into stir-fries, but when I ate out I often felt like I was entering hostile territory where friends and others wanted to ridicule my dietary choices. "Don't you want a big, juicy burger?" was practically a mantra. "Really? You don't eat meat? Good—more for me!" was another favorite. And then there's the asinine, "But what about the poor carrots?" This was the beginning of my period of misanthropy, which lasted for years. I looked at a lot of people with some level of disgust. I felt alienated, angry, burdened with understanding. I would explain, with great passion, how farm animals live day-to-day on factory farms, enduring lives far more miserable than we realize, and that their deaths are brutal and terrifying. If friends didn't choose to act on this new information immediately and boycott animal suffering, I'd lose some degree of respect for them. I couldn't help it. Although the movie was still years away at the time, it was like *The Matrix*, where Morpheus offers Neo a choice between two pills: A blue pill that would return him to his old life and a red pill that would allow him to learn the answers he seeks—or in this case, the truth, the real world—what lies beyond the routine facade. In my reality, anyone who didn't choose the red pill was choosing to be shallow and uncaring and willfully ignorant—all for the trivial pleasure of his or her taste buds.

Taking the Red Pill

I was fighting my fight virtually alone, without role models, without perspective. It would be years until I developed compassion for people who needed time with the new information. It would be years until I discovered that millions of people felt the exact same way I did, that local communities of people were working toward the same goals I was. These were people who had changed their lives like I was changing mine and they had some lessons to teach me about how to be an effective advocate.

As with many transformations and newly discovered passions, it can take a while to find your way, to refine your emotions and communicate with others in a way that will make a real difference. The more I saw that others weren't following my lead, the more exasperated and angry I became. I wore my impatience on my face and slathered my car and chest with bold messages: "Meat Is Murder! Fur Is Dead!" I was a bitter proselytizer, which was neither pretty nor effective. Let's just say I wasn't such a fun person to be around. But I had no examples of how to channel my energy in a constructive way—not yet.

The Horrible Bunny

A lbert Schweitzer was a theologian, philosopher, and Nobel Prize–winning vegetarian who urged us, "Think occasionally of the suffering of which you spare yourself the sight." This is, hands down, one of my favorite quotes. Our culture tells us to seek ease and indulgence, not to think critically about how our system works and live our lives accordingly. We push the uncomfortable truth away, shrugging, "Better not to think about it." We're taught that the days of American sacrifice are over and that unmitigated abundance with a low price tag is our birthright. We don't seem to want to look at the hidden price tag, no matter how high the moral, ethical, environmental, and health costs.

Schweitzer also said, "We must fight against the spirit of unconscious cruelty with which we treat the animals. Animals suffer as much as we do. True humanity does not allow us to impose such sufferings on them. It is our duty to make the whole world recognize it. Until we extend our circle of compassion to all living things, humanity will not find peace."

The Lucky Ones

One fall day in 2007, a little goat was found limping alone and terrified in Brooklyn's Prospect Park. Not knowing what else to do with him, local law enforcement turned him over to one of New York City's overcrowded dog and cat shelters, Animal Care and Control. We'd been on the ACC contact list for several years by then, since we were the closest farm animal shelter to New York City and, believe it or not, quite a few farm animals are found wandering the streets of NYC. The shelter called us and sent us pictures of the mystery goat, and we responded immediately.

Our best guess is that Albie had somehow escaped a live-kill market. Unbeknownst to most of its residents, New York City is home to almost a hundred such markets chock-full of chickens, rabbits, goats, sheep, and calves, penned and slaughtered right there on site. Customers can buy halal meat, slaughtered according to Islamic law, or kosher meat, slaughtered according to Jewish law—although never at the same place! These small, local markets are in some ways the opposite of factory farms, but they are by no means bastions of animal welfare and public health. Animals are strung up by their back legs and have their throats slits to "bleed out" without being rendered unconscious, causing animals to thrash and gasp for air for up to two minutes if not done correctly. Not the picture of humane, is it? And if you've just moved your hundred-chicken, twenty-goat, thirty-sheep killing operation into a defunct auto-body shop in Queens, ethical concerns and disease control may not be high on your list. Government regulations of the markets, when they even exist, are ambiguous and often ignored. So, along with raising serious ethical questions, the U.S. Department of Agriculture calls these disease incubators, among other things, the "missing link in the epidemiology of avian influenza."

We try to imagine the moment of escape for the animals who manage it. Were they just arriving and darted off during unloading? Were they being led from their pens, moments from slaughter? Was someone taking them home alive to slaughter at a celebration or religious gathering? We usually don't know for sure, but regardless, our primary concern is bringing them to safety.

The day after the initial phone call, a van rumbled down our driveway, carrying the precious cargo. I helped the driver unload a cage and set it gently on the grass, then knelt down to look inside. Pressed as far back as he could cowered a little white goat. I talked to him gently to lure him out. The pictures hadn't done justice to the depths of his problems: His mouth and nostrils were encrusted with cracking, oozing sores, evidence of a painful disease called orf, or sore mouth. It was the worst case I'd ever seen. He was also seriously underweight. And his little legs had deep impressions left by tight ropes or wire—a sign that he'd been hog-tied (all four legs tied together to make handling and transportation easier—and crueler). He was terrified and in pain, but I could see in his eyes that he was a gentle soul. So I named him after the wise, gentle, impeccably spoken, animal-loving Albert Schweitzer.

Orf is communicable to other animals and to humans (think of herpes sores, on steroids), so we prepared our back shed and surrounded it with a fenced-in area so that Albie could heal in isolation. It was the farthest point from other animals on the farm. Whenever we needed to treat him or wanted to spend time with him, we donned iso suits and gloves and dipped our shoes in a bleach solution. Then we'd sit down with the little goat, tend to his wounds, and comfort him.

It was no surprise that Albie was also rather emaciated. Orf makes chewing so painful that animals sometimes die of starvation; we needed to treat him right away. We dabbed his sores with healing salves and started him on supplements, and within about two weeks, the sores disappeared. His eating became a pleasure instead of a chore, and he grew more relaxed. Albie had begun to figure out that we were not there to hurt him, only to help him, and there was no need to be afraid.

The biggest issue, though, was what we discovered during our initial examination of him. The indentations on his legs from the wire hog ties looked serious but not serious enough to cause the amount of limping I noticed. With the help of Doug and our first paid animal caretaker, Robin, we laid Albie on his side to have a better look at the injured front leg. I noticed some dried blood around one of his front legs, so I brushed his shaggy white fur back with my gloved hand to have a better look. I gasped. The wire had caused a deep laceration that was hidden by his fur, and there was movement under the skin. Maggots! There must have been a hundred of them, eating away at what was once healthy tissue. I almost puked and cried at the same time. Poor baby—the wound had gone unnoticed at the ACC, and I couldn't imagine what those days must have felt like.

We immediately got to work, which wasn't easy because of his fear. The last time he had been turned over on his side was surely done roughly and ended with his legs painfully bound. Albie wiggled and protested every time we touched the area, occasionally crying out in pain. As gently as we could, we shaved the fur around the wound. Then we flushed it out repeatedly with saline and tweezed out the remaining maggots, a process that took close to half an hour. It was awful. The sound of a goat crying tears out your heart. It is the saddest, most earnest wailing that I've ever heard.

Once we'd gotten the wound as clean as we could, we wrapped it and started him on an antibiotic to stop the infection. The vet warned us right off the bat that Albie might lose the leg, but I wouldn't hear it. We followed instructions for treatment and hoped to give Albie a fighting chance. I knew that his life would change dramatically if he couldn't keep his leg. I feared he'd be slower than the rest of the herd, have trouble hunkering down to eat or graze, and would be exhausted by the effort of living on three legs.

But Albie's leg just wouldn't heal. Topical and oral antibiotics, herbal poultices, soaks, homeopathic remedies . . . we tried everything. Soon, though, we began to notice that his little hoof began to slough off, a sign that the tissue was becoming necrotic. X-rays showed just how bad the damage was: the bone had been affected, and even the strongest high-dose antibiotics weren't working. There was no reversing it. We chose to take a gamble and had the dead bone in his foot surgically removed, leaving him with only a partial hoof to stand on. This helped for a few months, but further X-rays showed that more of the bone was weak and crumbling from the previous infection. We talked to experts, including top-notch veterinarians at Cornell Veterinary Hospital, and realized that there was no alternative. It looked like there would soon be two amputees at the sanctuary.

I was heartbroken. I understood for the first time what my mother must have gone through when I was a kid, the profound sadness she must have felt when she faced the reality that my leg had to be amputated in order to save my life. Could there have been another way to stop the cancer from spreading? Maybe. But I looked back and understood that my mother and doctors felt they had no choice.

■ ■ ■ ■

Once Albie was safely through the amputation surgery and healing well, we turned ourselves to the next challenge: finding a way for him to walk on four legs.

Unlike dogs and cats, who can generally maneuver just fine on three legs, goats aren't anatomically designed to adjust easily to life as a tripod. They need the balance of limbs to lie down, stand up, graze, run, exercise, and socialize. As they get older, imbalance can put a great deal of stress on their spines. So once Albie's residual limb (aka "stump") had healed, I contacted my own prosthetist, Erik Tompkins, to see if he'd be willing to fit a goat. This was a request he had never heard, and it kind of blew his mind. But luckily, he's a cool guy and was game to give a nonhuman a go and, in fact, was totally up for the challenge. Erik came to the farm to meet his new patient, and then he got to work casting and measuring. He made a mold of Albie's stump and built a socket to its specifications, then lined it with comfortable padding. Next he added a metal support with a rubber stopper on the bottom that would give Albie traction in the grass and barn.

I couldn't wait for Albie's first fitting. So far, his adjustment had been awkward. He'd woken up one day to find he had lost a leg, and there was no way to explain the situation to him. He'd paw at the air, wondering why his phantom foot wasn't touching the ground. It must have been disorienting and uncomfortable. We were hopeful that this leg could get him closer to his old life.

A week or so later, the limb was ready, and we strapped it onto him one beautiful fall afternoon. I was ridiculously excited and optimistic, but Albie didn't get it. He cocked his head with such a puzzled look, you could imagine a cartoon bubble over his head that read, "What the #$@#?!" He immediately lifted this weird appendage in a sort of salute because he didn't want to put it down. I gently pushed his new leg toward the ground to show him he could prop himself up with it. After repeating the motion for him over and over again, he finally began to let the leg relax and put some weight on it.

The next hurdle was to actually walk with the leg. When he first gave that a try, he ended up alternating between hopping and dragging it along the grass, using no effort in his shoulder to pick it up and plant it down in a stepping motion. I hoped, unrealistically, to see him take to it immediately, but after a frustrating hour or so, we decided to give up for the day. We took the leg off to check his stump and make sure all was well. Then I remembered the months it took me to even hold my leg down post-amputation, because the blood flow ending abruptly caused throbbing and pain. I also remembered the further weeks it took me to be able to step down with my new artificial leg attached. It hurt like hell.

But Albie had had time to heal, and it was time to make it happen. Several days went by with daily sessions of strapping the leg on, getting Albie to put weight on it, then . . . GO! But he wouldn't. This was much harder than I ever imagined. Without verbal communication, instructing little Albie was ridiculously difficult. We'd stop our sessions when I could see he was tiring and when I became too frustrated. Ergh—if only we could explain! Patience, young Skywalker, patience!

Around day four, I came up with an idea. If actions speak louder than words, the action of luring with treats speaks loudest of all. That afternoon became a life lesson in the power of food. We moved all the other goats inside the barn so we wouldn't get bum-rushed, then led Albie out a side door. I slipped the leg onto him, held the "foot" to the ground, and then had Doug step in. We started with apple slices. Sure enough, he moved straight to Doug, drag-ging the leg all the way. I stopped him in his tracks, grabbed the leg and moved it for him—lifting with his shoulder, then stepping down. All his force was against me with every step as he fought to get to the sweet-smelling apples. Then, FINALLY—he got it. It was an Anne Sullivan–Helen Keller moment! He picked the leg up and took a few awkward steps, then dragged it again. I stopped him and mimicked the motion for him once again. By that time, we had let him eat the entire apple, so I chose to pull out the big guns: Alfalfa cubes, the crack cocaine of the ungulate world. Soon enough, after maybe a dozen attempts, there he was, awkward but walking—and quickly! He had to get to those alfalfa cubes. (These, by the way, are nothing more than dried, compressed alfalfa grass, but you would think they were Belgian truffles.)

It took time, just as it had for me, but eventually Albie found that he could indeed maneuver more comfortably with his prosthetic than he could without it. At first, we kept it on him for only a couple of hours a day. Often, we soon learned, he'd wiggle out of it, and we'd have to go search for it out in the pasture. But within a couple of weeks, he was using it to hobble around for hours at a time. We were so excited the first time we watched him lean to the ground to graze instead of kneeling lopsided.

Albie's is the kind of story that doesn't want to keep to itself, and the notion of an amputee sanctuary owner helping an amputee goat proved irresistible. Word spread to a *New York Times* reporter. Fernanda Santos called me one July afternoon, and she showed up, warm and enthusiastic, soon after, along with photographer Joyce Dopkeen. They were excited to meet Albie and tour the farm. Joyce was retiring, and at the end of our day together, she told me she couldn't have thought of a better story on which to end her long, storied photography career as the first female staff photographer at the *Times*.

A couple of days later, the phone rang very early in the morning. On the other end were Doug and his mom, Carole, who were both staring at the front page of that day's *Times* Metro section. Carole lives on Manhattan's Upper West Side, still in the same apartment where my husband grew up and where, coincidentally, he'd crashed the night before after a film-editing job. "Jenny!" Carole shouted. "We're looking at a huge picture of you and Albie!" And huge it was—the photo took up about half the page. None of us could believe it. "Hey," Doug said, "do we even *mention* his new leg on the website?" A mad scramble ensued, as often happens when things loom large at the expense of details. In the dark ages before Facebook and Twitter were widely used, it took a fair amount of technical knowledge to spread the word. "Nerd powers: Activate!" said Doug, and he was able to commandeer his mom's fax machine to scan the article in pieces, stitch them together in Photoshop, and upload the result to our home page. I knew I married him for a reason!

From there, the phone rang and rang, and our e-mail account seemed set to burst. We got calls from TV stations, literary agents, and reporters around the globe. We heard from people looking to volunteer and people who wanted to write checks. We had our busiest summer of visitors yet. That one article netted us $70,000 in donations—enough, at that time, to feed and care for the sanctuary's residents for three months solid, enough to help more animals in need. If I'd had known all this would happen just from showing a little leg . . . (cue snare drum: *ba-dum-bum*).

Speaking of, I did an unusual thing just before the photo shoot. Because of my level of activity, I need a high-tech, lightweight leg with carbon-fiber components. I still like to be able to slip on some skinny pants without odd cave-ins underneath, though, so having a leg-shaped cosmetic cover is normally my preference. But sometimes, and I knew this shoot would be one of those times, I choose to be Robo-Lady and flaunt my high-tech stuff. This article was going to partially feature my artificial leg, so I didn't want to be sporting my old stolen-off-a-mannequin look. If shock value would lead to awareness of our mission and organization, I was all for it. Fortunately, I had just had some work done on my leg and the "skin" had been removed, exposing the foam that hides the prosthesis's inner workings. Much to Erik Tompkins's dismay, I took a box cutter to the foam, revealing the stark carbon fiber form underneath. The photo certainly gets people's attention: a woman with a bionic-looking leg kissing a goat with only half a leg himself.

Visitors to the farm usually have no idea that there is anything different about me. Anyone who's ever worked on a farm knows that keeping your legs covered is smart, so I usually wear pants or jeans. I do walk with a slight limp, but most don't notice it. I discovered early on conducting tours that it was better that way because people (especially children) tend to pay so much attention to my leg that they might not hear what I'm saying. This is my only opportunity to share with visitors how farmed animals live and die to end up on our plates. I hope that by sharing the truth, others might come to the same decisions I have. So I keep my leg on the down-low . . . until I need it.

Generous and much-needed contributions aside, I received countless letters from inspired and touched readers. "Bless you," they'd say, "you're doing God's work!" And, "What an inspiration!" You'd think I was Mother Teresa. The unexpected outpouring, and seeing the name of our fledgling nonprofit in *THE New York Times*, made me feel exhilarated and oh so thankful.

Best of all, though, was the change the piece created in people. Before reading about Albie, most people had never seen animals like him as anything but "livestock." Now they were revisiting their assumptions. They'd heard of paralyzed dogs being custom-fitted with carts to help them get around, but that followed the usual course of dog-as-family-member thinking that much of our society subscribes to. But this story was something different. Are goats worth that much trouble? Goats are routinely raised for their milk and meat around the country, and goat meat, believe it or not, is the most consumed meat in the world. But Albie's story turned him into an individual: he had a name, he was loved, he wouldn't be *used* for anything, and he had been through an awful ordeal. He became the rock star of the sanctuary overnight.

I discovered my passion for animal rights practically the moment I stepped onto the U of L campus. By my third year, though, I discovered another passion: film. I took a photography class that engrossed me, and soon after I picked up an old 8mm film camera and started shooting. I was especially drawn to cinematography, the visual manifestation of explorations and ideas. I wanted more experiences in my life, new experiences, and film could be a door to those. I wasn't interested in working on blockbusters; those wouldn't broaden my horizons the way something like National Geographic would, so I wanted to work on documentaries. But I couldn't gain a foothold in anything like that if I didn't look beyond the Louisville horizon right away. I wanted to go film school.

At that time, besides one trip to Florida with my friend Cindy when I finished all my chemo treatments, the farthest I had been outside Kentucky was a little town my mother would drive us to in Brown County, Indiana, where we would feast on homemade apple butter and visit the John Dillinger Wax Museum. Now I was thinking about living, working, and studying in another state, potentially far from home. To soften the blow, I chose Chicago. It was a large enough city to make me feel I was heading somewhere significant and to house a relatively inexpensive film school—Columbia

College—but it was also a relative spitting distance from home: a five-hour drive. I could go home on weekends to stave off home-sickness when my schedule allowed.

Columbia accepted me, though I'd need two more years of college there to finish my degree, and I had already been through three. Oh, well. I got my hands on a Chicago paper, pored over the classifieds, and found a cheap apartment near the college. On leaving day, Boogie and I said an emotional good-bye to my mom. "I'm gonna miss you so much," I told her. "Who am I gonna come home and spew all my venomous rage to?" I laughed. She was always so patient when I'd tell her the latest animal atrocities I'd read or heard about. "Who's gonna cook for me, Mom?" Yes, pathetic. I really never cooked for myself. I've never lived down the time I opened a can of cream of mushroom soup and read the cooking instructions to add one can of water. "Do you think they mean this can?" I asked, thinking that a "can" might be a formal measurement. My mother and sister almost died laughing.

"I'm going to miss you, too, baby girl." Ugh. I hated it when she called me this (she still does). She was terrified just thinking about me in Chicago. "Don't ever leave your door unlocked, and carry your purse real tight. Don't answer the door to a stranger. . . ." My parting gift was a keychain-size bottle of Mace.

Finally, Boogie and I started our journey north, made it to my new apartment, and moved my boxes and her litter box into our new digs with the help of my sister and some friends. Boogie was excited about the sunny bay window, and I was excited to have my own place. Neither of those things, though, kept us from heading home as often as I could for the first few months I was there. Lord, I was homesick! Nothing in Chicago was familiar, and that was a double-edged sword. Only Boogie provided me with family and a connection to home.

Navigating the city, bill paying, grocery shopping, cooking . . . everything involved a learning curve, school most of all. Columbia College was a bustling hub of creative hipsters who majored in some form of the arts: dance, music, theater, film and animation, fashion. Instead of Biology 101 and English 102, I was taking Film Tech I and Intro to Documentary Production. I dove in, mastering sophisticated cameras and equipment, learning the art of composition, of sound. At times I felt like the resident small-town transplant, pushing out of my bubble but feeling a little culturally and intellectually behind others. I'd hear myself say "y'all" and "ain't," and other students would giggle and poke fun. I started trying to suppress some of that Southern speech. And I hadn't studied the who's who of film. "I'm more drawn to the subtly antiauthoritarian aspects of Kieslowski's oeuvre than the more overt political work of, say, Lumet," a fellow student might proclaim. I still hadn't even seen *Citizen Kane*. Oh, the shame!

At the end of my first year, I directed and produced a black-and-white film that directly challenged that small-town bubble. It was an arty take on homosexuality that cast it in a positive light. Back when I started college, I had looked at homosexuality as a sin, as deviancy, because that's what I was brought up to believe. I was embarrassed by my former views and wanted to go full-throttle challenging those beliefs. My film even featured a full-on passionate kiss between two men. The film ended up being selected as one of the ten Best of the Fest films at the Columbia College Chicago film festival and landed me as "one to watch" among the students.

In Chicago, I completely let go of any self-consciousness

regarding my leg. I'd walk along the Lake Michigan beaches clad only in a bikini, no jeans or towel around my waist. I'd watch the many faces check me out: Men's eyes would travel from my chest to my legs, a look of appreciation changing to one of puzzlement or embarrassment as they froze on my leg, then traveled back up to my eyes to catch me staring back. I'd smile and just carry on, choosing to banish any more thoughts.

One summer day, my blonde bombshell friend Kymm and I were lying on blankets on the beach, rubbing ourselves down with suntan lotion. Kymm had come up from Louisville for a long weekend, and we were both eager to work on our tans.

"Check those guys out," I said, pointing at a group of gorgeous men playing volleyball.

"They are HOT," she agreed.

"They're not speaking English—do you think they're Spanish?" I asked. That was about the extent of my knowledge of other cultures.

Soon, they started amusing themselves by watching us watch them. When they finally took a break, one of them came over. He'd seen me, he'd seen the leg, and he still came over. Not to talk to the blonde on my left with four natural limbs, but to me, with three . . . and a half. I was shocked. This was a first.

In every previous relationship, since it was difficult to tell that there was anything different about me at first (unless I was wearing shorts), I'd had to decide when and how to tell the guy I was out on a date with what I was like "below the knee." Once I had, unfortunately, the energy would sometimes change. I never had someone run for the door, but I had some relationships fizzle out soon after, and there was always the question in my mind as to why. But

Marcelo—who turned out to be Brazilian, not Spanish, and in fact it had been Portuguese I was hearing—knew up front. There was no coming out: I was out. And he was in. A couple of days later, he and I went out for dinner. That date lasted almost three years. Suddenly, I wasn't heading home on the weekends as much.

Being out on my own meant I could now surround myself with like-minded souls and shed some of the indoctrinations that defined me as a young person. I was beginning to understand that the church saw animals as lesser-than, as beings here for us to exploit and have "dominion over." I now saw animals as beings we shared the world with. The church saw other religious systems, along with homosexuality, atheism, and premarital sex, as sins. I now saw them as nobody else's damn business.

This was blasphemy. Raised as I was in the bosom of a Southern Baptist family and community, separating myself was nothing short of a struggle. I wanted to remain respectful to my family and of my roots, but I was realizing that the world was full of choices about religion—sects, denominations, and intensities. Before I got to college, I hadn't explored religion much outside our sect of Christianity. When I took a religion course, I felt small-minded by my limited knowledge of the subject, considering how deeply entrenched in it I was. The sheer number of other faiths astounded me, and that knowledge made me refashion my own faith. I didn't stop believing in a divine presence, but I did start to believe that Jesus, Allah, the Buddha, Jah, Krishna, and all other deities are just different names for God, and that what God means to people has many variations.

My mother did *not* like to hear me talk about my new nondenominational slant. She panicked. "Your soul will be lost, Jenny!"

The Horrible Bunny

"How can you be worried about my soul when there's so much evil out there?"

"But the Bible is the word of God—have you lost your faith?"

Conversations with my grandparents were daggers in their backs. My family despaired that I wouldn't see them in the afterlife if I didn't keep Jesus Christ as our Lord and savior in my heart. And here I was questioning and—in their minds, disregarding—everything I'd been brought up to believe: deeply ingrained tenets. It was painful for me, too, to disengage from that, to deny Jesus and the Bible—it was like denying a piece of myself. But learning about other religions made me see that one needn't have that philosophy of domination over other living beings. Now I look at that philosophy as speciesism: "a failure, in attitude or practice, to accord any nonhuman being equal consideration and respect."

As for the God I grew up with, why did he so readily allow apathy and antipathy toward animals? How could he allow animals, human and nonhuman, to suffer to this extent? Why the language about "dominion"? And why was our use of animals never discussed in church? I was exploring the idea that organized religion led, or at least allowed, people to think we can criminally exploit and torture other living beings. People of Abrahamic faiths—Christians, Jews, Muslims—often argue that eating meat is "the will of God." I would hope that if they knew the modern-day horrors of factory farming, they might agree that is not what God intended. But deeply rooted ideology has allowed cruel farming practices to go unchallenged. However, there is no commandment to eat meat and no prohibition of adopting a vegetarian diet. To live a good life, then, wouldn't we want to take a stand against the systematized cruelty and deprivation that animals endure?

I couldn't believe in a system like that, no matter what it meant for my past, my family, and my existence. I only wanted to believe in a compassionate God, and that's exactly what I still do. I have my own personal religion in which God includes animals in "Thou shall not murder" and looks at our mindless consumption of them as not only unnecessary, but, unless there are absolutely no other options, unethical. I am comforted by the idea that if there is an afterlife for us, there has to be one for the animals, too. One where we are able to see and understand the wrongs we have committed on this earth and against animals whom we have used, abused, exploited, deprived, and murdered. In my idea of afterlife, all of those victims live the most blissful life imaginable alongside us. It may sound simple and childish, but it's a hope, or rather a faith, that helps me sleep at night.

But we humans are nothing if not complicated. It's hard to believe now, but when I first moved to Chicago, I found a job waiting tables at a Bennigan's. That's right: a baby-back-ribs-serving corporate restaurant chain. There I was serving up beef fajitas and chicken tenders, one plate after another. I was far less oblivious about the role I was playing than the teenage Jenny selling Big Macs, though, so it was agonizing to smile while I set down those plates. As an ethical vegetarian—one who chooses to be so not just for health reasons—I felt like a complete hypocrite. But my beliefs weren't as fully formed as they are now, and a gal needs to earn a living! In order to live on my own and pay the rent while going to school full-time, I had to have a job with flexible hours and plenty of them, and I knew very little about the city. Bennigan's meant a paycheck, good tips, and a walk right down the block from Columbia College. And a really dorky uniform.

The Horrible Bunny

Luckily, a coworker there soon introduced me to the Chicago Diner. "You're a vegetarian and you don't know about the Diner?"

"I don't have any vegetarian friends here yet—this is the first I'm hearing about it!"

"Well, it's a veg restaurant on the other side of town, and it's been around for years. It's a happening place—you should check it out."

The Diner opened its doors in 1983 ("Meat-free since '83") and was a swinging hot spot by the time I got to town in the early '90s. It was an oasis for us weirdos who believed wings are for flying, not frying. Hippies and hipsters, musicians and macrobiotics, students and animal rights activists crammed into its battered wooden booths. Sarah McLaughlin and the Pixies piped through the speakers, and writers scribbled at the Formica counter, cups of bancha tea cooling at their elbows. For the first time in my life, I was surrounded by My People. I didn't feel strange or uncomfortable or alienated, I felt welcomed. And finally, a restaurant where I could order anything on the menu!

I met my first vegans at the Diner, and tasted my first vegan desserts. The menu burst with new flavors. Tempeh? Seitan? What the hell are those? And here was tofu outside my mom's well-meaning but less-than-gourmet hands. I couldn't get enough of the menu. I didn't love everything, but I loved a lot.

At the time, vegans struck me as pretty Out There—a little too radical. I followed the notion that misguides many vegetarians. I remember talking to Joan, who was vegan and so cool with her short hair, no makeup, and unshaved armpits. She was the Joni Mitchell of my scene. "If you're not killing the animal, what's the problem?" I asked her.

"You'd be surprised at how much misery goes into the making of milk and eggs," she replied. But for some reason, I didn't take her seriously—it seemed more like personal militancy than a general philosophy to take seriously. I wish she had really sat me down and talked to me about how the animals in the dairy and egg industries actually have worse lives than their meat-producing counterparts; that they also become meat, but have a longer and more miserable life before the slaughterhouse. I think I shut down the conversation before it got there because I didn't want to know—and didn't think I could ever enjoy eating again with so many limitations. It would take me years to learn that and to discover the cruel truth behind dairy and eggs.

One night at work, I set a cup of coffee in front of a woman sitting alone, a sheaf of papers spread out in front of her. The PETA letterhead on one of her documents caught my eye. On my way back to her with her soup, I mustered the courage to clear my throat and ask, "Do you work for PETA?"

"I sure do," she said.

I was in awe; I got the same feeling in my gut you would if you met a rock star—to me, people working in and dedicating their lives to animal advocacy are the real rock stars. "You mean you actually work for them?"

She laughed. "I'm in town to organize the annual fur march."

"What's that?" I put down my tray.

"It's a protest on North Michigan Avenue in front of some of the big department stores that sell fur," she explained.

I told her I was in film school and would love to help out in any way I could, and by the time I brought Cam her check an hour later,

The Horrible Bunny

I'd agreed to film the protest for her and for a documentary assignment for school. It was a win-win.

I couldn't have been more excited. Before that night, I'd been too busy adjusting to life as a Chicago resident, full-time film student, and full-time waitress to focus on promoting animal rights causes, but now an opportunity to get involved was there for the taking. This was a chance to do more than just abstain from meat; it was a chance to get involved with a high-profile organization that worked specifically for animal rights.

The demonstration itself took place two days later. The streets were packed, and I was beyond exhilarated. I'd done man-on-the-street filming before for class assignments, so I felt pretty comfortable getting reactions and brief interviews among the demonstrators, onlookers, and even a cop. I followed the activists as they brandished signs depicting horrifying images of animals caught in traps, living in tiny cages, and being skinned or anally electrocuted—gruesome. PETA really knew what they were doing. The event was organized and dramatic, complete with slick leaflets, signs, and banners and a nice crowd of enthusiastic, informed demonstrators.

Things got going when a group of solemn-faced, black-cloaked mourners joined us at the corner of Grand and Michigan about twenty minutes into the walk. Twelve of them hefted two wooden coffins onto their shoulders and began to trudge down the Miracle Mile. PETA had put the word out that they needed donated fur coats, old and new, from whoever was willing to let them go. As we made our way toward the major department store area, bystanders placed twenty or so in the passing caskets. Beaver, rabbit, fox, chinchilla, mink: I looked at the coats and wondered how many animals had suffered and died for each of them, all for the sake of fashion and status.

Occasional heckling further charged the atmosphere. "Don't you have anything better to do?" one man yelled. "Get a job!" shouted another. "In fact, get a life!" One guy was a little more original, at least: "I'm buying my wife a fur coat for Christmas!" Even this early in my activism days, I'd already made a solid observation on this kind of behavior: Faced with uncomfortable truths that involve their participation on some level, people can become very defensive. I would later attend a circus protest where I was pummeled by the fury of people who didn't want their comfortable assumptions challenged. On that occasion, I remember retaliating with a litany of profanities and facts about the miserable lives of circus animals. They just laughed and rolled their eyes, one telling me to shut up, another telling me to go f**k myself. Later I felt bad cursing and screaming in front of children who thought they were just going for a fun afternoon to see the circus. I told myself afterward that I needed to control the urge to lash out. It just wasn't effective. Not only did it wreck me physically and mentally, it made people stand taller in their positions, since it gave them something to legitimately have a problem with: the angry, screaming protesters themselves.

Because I videoed the fur protest, I was a bit distanced from the interactions between the protesters and the agitators trying to get a rise out of them. Most protesters just ignored them as they belted out chants like "No blood for vanity!" I did, though, witness the occasional middle finger make an appearance.

Our funeral procession finally stopped in front of Saks Fifth

Avenue, one of the stores that sold fur (and still does). Protesters set the coffins down in a row on the wide sidewalk and, as some volunteers began passing out leaflets to people entering and exiting the store, others lit matches and set the furs ablaze in their caskets. The smell of burning hair cut into the air, and smoke billowed wildly. When it cleared, I zoomed in on the fire, then out on the faces of chanting activists and surprised onlookers. I had no idea what would happen next. Simply put, this was the most exciting thing I'd ever been part of. The protesters continued their march, now in a wide circle around the burning coffins, still shouting chants at Saks.

The police wasted little time. I followed them with my lens as they stalked over.

"Who's in charge?" one of them said, waving smoke away.

Cam, my friend from the Chicago Diner, stepped forward, her face impassive except for a glint in her eye. "I am."

"Turn around."

Another officer yanked the bullhorn from her hands and spun her around to click on the cuffs. I was near breathless as I filmed her being shoved into the back of the cop car, news camera operators who had since arrived doing the same. Some of the protesters followed her to the precinct a few blocks away, waving signs, chanting, and leafleting. We stayed there for some time, but when it became obvious her bail would take a while to post, I packed up the camera. I was anxious to get the lowdown from Cam the next day. In the coming week, I edited the footage and put together some scenes. I couldn't wait to send it to her.

Unlike the blocked and scripted film and video work I'd done in the past, this was real life. It was grassroots activism and work with people who cared like I did, working toward an important cause. Even my classmates were excited by the resulting piece, and as I screened it for them and listened to the resulting discussion, I could see firsthand how effective film could be. I was hooked.

So I didn't stop there. I wanted to do more, but in order to do so, PETA wanted me to prove my allegiance to the cause and my bravery in general. They'd planned another protest, this time at an advertising awards ceremony taking place at a fancy hotel right in Chicago. Gillette, notorious for their animal experiments, was winning the grand award for a TV ad campaign that used cutting-edge face-morphing technology.

PETA set up the protest carefully and sent press releases to local media. By the time the event began, while protesters held up signs and shouted from the opposite side of the street, I was already in the hotel cocktail lounge with another activist and a lawyer for PETA. Then, while invited guests were out in the lobby sipping cocktails before entering the main event room, we snuck down to the basement where my costume had been planted earlier. I slipped myself into a horrible-looking bunny suit that came from PETA headquarters, stepping into the giant feet and sliding on the enormous rabbit head. Its eyes had been made to look like those of a bunny undergoing Draize testing. As I mentioned before, this is a notoriously cruel eye-irritation test during which experimenters drip or smear chemicals into an animal's eyes while he is immobilized. Typically the rabbit is immobilized in a metal box with only his head sticking out, leaving his eyes painfully swollen, irritated, and bordered with droopy red, hairless folds of skin. The costume head looked awful—and perfect.

The other activist helped me hang the sign around my neck that read, "Gillette Tortures Animals. Shame on Gillette!" as we stepped onto the staff elevator. I was scared to death! We had two floors up to go. We hoped that no one would call the elevator in the meantime—we didn't want to get busted while security, due to the protest outside, was swarming the place.

The first-floor light lit up, and before we could panic, the elevator doors opened and in walked—I kid you not—Tony Bennett! I couldn't believe my chemically burnt eyes. *The* Tony Bennett stepped right on with a bodyguard, who immediately pulled out his walkie-talkie after reading my sign. The star looked surprised, and his flashy grin turned to a look of concern as he stared at the grotesque face of the rabbit costume. Then his eyes traveled down to the sign around my neck. "Oh, goodness, I had no idea."

"Well, here, take a pamphlet and read all about it!" my fellow activist exclaimed, and at that moment, the doors opened to the second floor and out I ran, chanting, "Gillette tortures animals! Shame on Gillette!!!" I was having trouble keeping my bunny head on straight, desperate to see where I was going through the eye holes as I made my way into the crowd. I caught a glimpse of attendees, their mouths wide open in shock, darting away from me. My partner followed, handing out literature on Gillette's crimes while chanting along with me.

Within a minute, I felt a forceful hand grab my shoulder, and security guards pushed me to the ground facedown and pulled my paws behind me. They fumbled to put handcuffs on the bunny suit but had to give up. They wanted me out of there quickly, so two of them escorted me back to the elevator and removed my rabbit head. I had been given five hundred dollars to stash in my shoe in case I got arrested, but fortunately, they escorted me and the other activist outside and released us where other protesters stood. The lawyer stood by to witness the whole thing and protect us in case of trouble. Cheers and applause from the crowd heightened the moment but pissed off security. "The next one of you who enters the hotel will be arrested!" one of them barked. I'd gotten lucky but was shaking in my bunny feet for the rest of the day. I felt incredibly proud. I had passed the test—at least this one.

Soon after, while I was still between semesters, I got a call from Cam, who asked me to go on another assignment. I soon found myself touching down on the tarmac in Fargo, North Dakota.

Premarin was a drug I had never heard of, but I learned from the investigator who met my plane in Fargo that hundreds of thousands of women across the country were turning to this prescribed hormone treatment during menopause. Pregnant horses, scientists had found, spill great concentrations of hormones into their urine, and the name Premarin says it all: The drug comes from the piss of pregnant mares. But how to capture the urine in the amounts needed for all these women? Premarin farms were a brand-new form of factory farm originating in Manitoba, Canada, where the drug company giant Wyeth Ayerst (now owned by Pfizer) is located. The business was lucrative and demand was high, so farms started popping up everywhere in Manitoba's neighbor to the south, North Dakota. These miserable facilities confine the mares to narrow stalls six to seven months at a time, collecting their urine with a crude apparatus and tubing fastened between their legs. Since every drop means profit, there is no going out to pasture for these horses. They are confined day in and day out, standing on hard concrete floors and allowed very little water in order to increase the concentration of estrogens in their urine. This water deprivation often leads to liver and kidney disease and keeps the mares in a constant state of thirst. Their foals are taken away, usually before weaning, and sold at auctions. Many are purchased cheaply for horse meat to ship overseas where there is a market for it. Then the mothers are artificially inseminated to start the whole process over again.

I spent days and traveled many miles, driving from place to place looking for access to one of the farms. My travel companion, I'll call her Anna, was an undercover investigator who was in disguise in case she was seen at one of the facilities. She wouldn't even tell ME her real name. Anna had obtained jobs at several of the farms to document the horrifying conditions these horses lived and died in, but her assignment was too important to get caught videotaping or taking photos. So they sent me in to get video. Anna knew the locations, the cars owned by the workers, and the doors that might be left unlocked. After visiting four farms over the course of several days, we were finally able to get into the last one in North Dakota before Canada. We were prepared to drive into Canada to other locations if we needed to, but luckily, we didn't.

It was dark outside, and one lonely car sat a distance away by the farmer's home. I grabbed my backpack and readied my camera. We parked down the road and snuck through a field to reach the back of a dimly lit building. The back door was open a crack, and we crouched by the door, listening for human steps or voices. When we felt that the coast was clear, we quietly slid the door open and crept in, allowing time for our eyes to adjust. My hands shook as I reached into my bag and pulled out my camera, the smell of urine and feces assaulting my eyes and nose. I flipped on the camera light and steadied myself as I focused on the horror in front of me. About one hundred horses stood, row after row, stall after stall, branded with numbers on their rears, feces caked along their legs. This was their existence. I tried to fight back tears, but they streamed down anyway. I checked to make sure my image stabilization function was on because my hands were shaking so badly. I moved slowly down an aisle, capturing the mares' narrow stalls, the urine tubes, the sores between their legs from the hard plastic collection apparatus. The mares looked as scared as I did. I made sure to film their faces, hoping the viewer could look into their eyes and see their misery.

That footage was the first video ever taken inside a Premarin farm. The news package made its debut in Canada, Germany, the United Kingdom, and the United States, and is still accessible on YouTube and on PETA's website in a video narrated by Mary Tyler Moore. I couldn't have been more proud, but whenever I look at that footage my heart sinks. I wish that I could have cut all their tethers and set them free, and the thought of doing that ran through my mind the entire time I was there filming. But had we done so, we might have gotten caught and our footage confiscated, and that wouldn't have done us or the mares any good.

I had other assignments that year, some successful, some not. I secretly videotaped at a circus where elephants were routinely poked and hit with bullhooks; I tried but failed to gain access to a primate laboratory; and I had easier tasks, like documenting a

The Horrible Bunny

protest outside a retail furrier and organizing a circus protest back in Louisville.

Eventually, PETA offered me a job heading up its film and video department. I was thrilled with what the job offered—the chance to combine my two passions to work in film and animal rights. But the job would have me primarily archiving, making dubs (video duplications), and putting together video press kits. I would no longer be out on the front lines, and I just wasn't ready to settle into a staff position yet.

5

....

Take Two

I f you were going to a Halloween party dressed as an elf or a genie, imagine the shoes you would wear—the kind with upward-curling toes. That shape is what Louise the sheep's back hoof resembled. It was so overgrown from lack of trimming that it curled upward and around, hitting her shin. This was just one example of how her basic health care had been neglected. Domesticated cows, goats, horses, and other hooved animals who live exclusively on grass pasture all require trimming since they don't wear down their hooves traveling long distances on a variety of terrains (as would their wild counterparts). But Louise did not come from a big ranch where she could be lost in the herd; she was being raised at a run-down local farm with just a few dozen sheep.

Here in the Hudson Valley, and all over New York state, apple season is a big deal. Second only to Washington, New York produces more than three billion apples annually, and thousands of migrant workers are brought in to help the harvest. A major portion of the lamb farm's revenue was providing meat for the workers. And that's where Louise's story begins: A blob of wool was spotted in the snow by a man—let's call him Bob—driving by the "fresh lamb" sign during an extreme cold snap. It turned out to be Louise, and she was lying on her side, frozen to the ground. There was no adequate shelter for any of the animals, but Louise was weak and injured, unable to bear her own weight and huddle together with others for warmth. Upon inquiry, Bob learned that the farmer assumed she was nearly dead, and wasn't willing to take any action to save her. When Bob asked if he would be willing to part with her, the farmer said, "Be my guest."

Bob brought Louise home and warmed her by the fire. During the next several months, he lovingly helped her get her strength back and she started to walk again, but he wasn't equipped to deal with a farm animal long term. Almost six months later, the farmer got wind that Louise might have survived, and demanded to have her back, or get payment. We often hear this, almost like a punch line to a bad joke: Farmer X wants money for an animal he abused or left for dead months prior. Bob needed to relocate her before things went pear-shaped, and guess who got the phone call?

When Louise arrived here we saw evidence of problems beyond her feet. She'd lost half of her ear to frostbite; she was very underweight; her skin had a weird infection; and even though it was the end of summer, she'd not been sheared and her wool was matted and dreadlocked. To top it off, Louise's tail had been docked more severely than I'd ever seen—to the point where there wasn't even a nub indicating where her tail should be. Such tail mutilation is, heartbreakingly, a common practice in the industry, supposedly for the sake of hygiene and, in the case of lambs, avoidance of fly strike, a painful condition caused by blowflies.

Take Two

On my tours I often ask people to imagine drawing a picture of a sheep, and wouldn't they bestow it with a little bunny-rabbit tail? That's how we've come to think of sheep tails. But sheep aren't born that way. Then I point out our sheep who have their naturally long, bushy tails, and those who don't. At the sanctuary we'll sometimes find a sheep with a poopy tail and—go figure—a wet, warm rag or shearing the fleece around their behinds and tail will pretty much take care of that little problem. However, at a large ranch with hundreds if not thousands of sheep, it's much cheaper to dock all tails than to pay enough workers to notice.

This is one condition the industry *does* care about, not because of the discomfort, naturally, but because of the potential loss of their product, the wool. The docking "operations," which involve a hot blade or a rubber band fitted tightly around the tail until it becomes necrotic and falls off, are excruciating and conducted without anesthesia. Animals often suffer infections and chronic pain. The American Veterinary Medical Association's Animal Welfare Division says docking should be "avoided whenever possible" because of the "pain and distress" and "considerable discomfort" it causes. The organization suggests using shearing and topical medicines instead. But few farmers want to do something labor-intensive when they can opt for an easier method, no matter how painful, and there are no laws restricting said practices.

Louise's tail we couldn't replace, but getting her walking comfortably was within our reach. We deduced that an injury to her ankle caused that particular hoof to be so profoundly overgrown that her tendon had actually stretched to accommodate the misalignment. Now, after a proper hoof trim, the foot still pointed in the wrong direction. Compared with humans, sheep have an extra joint in their legs. This is the best way I can describe it: Imagine your ankle bent so that your foot is pointing straight up and you're walking on the back of your heel. Uncomfortable, right?

Fortunately, our local vet had experience in this area, and he recommended a brace to hold Louise's leg in the correct alignment. She hated this. It was essentially a fiberglass cast like you'd use for a broken leg, and between her skin infection, the heat of the late-summer days, and the need to protect the cast from rain with an uncomfortable-looking plastic bag, she was miserable.

The good news was that after about six weeks the brace had done its job: The tendon had shrunk to the point where her muscles could hold the leg in the proper position, and she could walk with only a minor limp. We were thrilled! Given all the difficulties we'd seen with Albie and his leg, we had been skeptical during Louise's time in the cast.

The most remarkable thing was that, throughout it all, Louise was a trouper. Unlike many animals who arrive at the sanctuary terrified of humans, she liked people. Really liked them. And all the attention, snacks, and constant handling increased her friendliness exponentially. Nowadays, while Louise likes being out with her flock, she really goes out of her way to seek out people, and, I mean, she loves people. She'll walk up to just about anyone and lean her head against their body or put her face right up to yours, if it's available. If no one is nearby when she's jonesing for a cuddle, she stands at the fence and bleats the saddest bleat you've ever heard. There is no tragedy tragic enough to justify such a bleat. I am unable to resist this, of course; the trick works every time and I'll endlessly scratch her behind her one perfect ear, and then her other half ear, just as perfect in a different way because it reminds us of where she came from.

Sometimes when I'm giving a farm tour and we go into the pasture with the sheep, I talk about how our culture views this species. We call people "sheep" when we want to portray them as mindless followers or when referring to a person lacking intelligence or common sense. But it makes sense for prey animals to stick together. If nature is about survival, safety in numbers is the smartest course for herd animals. And when you live with sheep and have gained their trust, it doesn't take long to see their varied personalities—especially if they know you. Sheep can recognize individual human and sheep faces and remember them for years. We get to know them and their unique qualities: Celia's nurturing, Louise's affection cravings, Mal's shyness, and Devlin's goofiness . . . each is an individual.

■ ■ ■ ■

B oogie and I moved back to Louisville about a year after college. Finding paid freelance work just out of film school was tough in Chicago, a city with so much competition. Moving out of titles such as "Production Assistant," basically a glorified gofer, would take a while. I needed to find work in my field that would utilize and pay me for my new skills. I decided to see if I could break into my hometown's smaller production scene. It was comforting to be back in familiar surroundings and with old friends, but I knew that Louisville would just be a stopping place, a place to build my resume.

After only a few months back in Louisville, I figured out that the production management end of things made more sense for me than cinematography. For one thing, it was incredibly difficult to break into camera work, and when you do break in, you typically have to start at the bottom. That entry-level work involves a lot of grueling equipment-schlepping. As much as I'd adjusted to my prosthetic and remained fit, some jobs in film/TV production were harder on me than others. Still, I tried to keep my leg a secret. I worried that all those underling schlep jobs would be closed to me, that heavy lifting was too much a part of the job for crews to take a chance on a "gimp." I tested my theory when I worked as a production assistant on a Kentucky Lotto commercial. When someone mentioned my slight limp, I responded truthfully that the fit on my prosthetic at the time wasn't quite right. From then on, the production manager would tell me not to worry about helping with physical tasks. I was determined to show them I could do it, so I helped out anyway. But as much as I tried to hide it, that choice led to some real pain and chafing on my residual limb. This was the mid-nineties, and prosthetics have come a long way since. Now, luckily, I rarely have such problems.

For another thing, camera work was a very male-dominated field back then. I knew only one female cinematographer, and I knew it had taken her a long time to establish relationships and prove herself to be not just capable but talented as well. I didn't feel I could afford to throw another stumbling block beyond disability—my gender—in front of me.

94

Take Two

The production management end of things was a pleasure for a detail-oriented multitasker like me. And while there was plenty of running around, about the heaviest thing I had to schlep was a clipboard. I managed to net some real experience in Louisville. I worked on some indie films, including my first feature film, *Lawn Dogs*, and later *Nice Guys Sleep Alone*. I also started work on a fascinating project with producer/director Mark Reese, baseball legend Pee Wee Reese's son: a documentary about the Beat generation.

While that project, sadly, didn't get off the ground, I did get a tattoo out of it. In the course of my research, I read a biography of Jack Kerouac, whose colorful, artsy, nomadic life wowed me. I read that his family's ancestral shield held the motto *"Aimer, Travailler et Souffrir"* (Love, Work, and Suffer). Those succinct words epitomized everything I felt as I tried to find my way in the world. That became my motto. When the documentary fell through, I went down to New Orleans to visit my sister, who was working as a nurse there. For my twenty-fifth birthday, Loren paid for the tattoo so I could immortalize Kerouac's words on my back in "tramp stamp" fashion. But of course this was 1995—before there were enough lower-back tattoos to warrant such a complimentary moniker. I consider myself a tramp-stamp pioneer.

Tattoos aside, I was disappointed to lose the only exciting documentary work I could find in Louisville. I remembered the kinds of projects I'd dreamed about, the ones that spurred me to go to film school in the first place, and they weren't commercials for Super-America gas stations or Papa John's Pizza.

I knew Boston was a hub for documentary production and that the mother ship of all public television, WGBH, was there, where *NOVA, Frontline, American Experience*, and other highly respected documentary programs were produced. Of course, this meant yet another move. But four years in Chicago had taught me confidence. And this time, I wasn't moving solo-plus-cat: I was with my new husband, Andy, a musician who was also excited about a move out of Louisville—although we'd both miss it terribly. We were young, Andy twenty-nine, me twenty-seven, but we were adults, and we were eager to plant ourselves firmly in our chosen fields of interest.

We settled into one of the few Boston neighborhoods we could afford, Allston, and began our new East Coast lives. Boogie seemed to be settling in happily, too, and on weekends she and I would go to a park near the water. I'd put a body harness on her and attach a leash, which she hated, and we'd lie on a blanket, which she loved (and made the dreaded leash worth it). She'd creep around with her belly low to the ground, exploring the blanket's vicinity, and I'd watch the hip urbanite joggers look at me like I was a crazy cat lady.

Almost right away, I found the kind of work I'd been looking for since I began studying film. Though it meant descending a few rungs on the ladder, these new gigs were documentaries and important stepping-stones. I knew that I'd rather be a production assistant for WGBH in Boston than a production manager for a bank commercial in Louisville. And early on, I landed a great gig working on a show for the long-running PBS series *NOVA*.

When that was over, I stayed at WGBH to work on several local shows. The buildings bustled with production. I'd meet people from *Antiques Roadshow*, *This Old House*, and *American Experience* in the lunchroom or during station-wide gatherings, and kids from *Zoom* would run screaming down the halls singing their theme song, "We're gonna zoom, zoom, zoom, a-zoom" (which brought back childhood memories of my sister and me singing and dancing along to the show). Our office was right next to one of my favorite NPR shows, *The World*. I loved the energy, the enthusiasm, the sophistication . . . and the progressive lunchroom, which, along with the one next door at Harvard (yes, *that* Harvard), offered lots of vegetarian options.

Only problem was, mobility was tough—and not the physical kind. The climb to the higher-level positions was steep and competitive. I could move more quickly, I realized, through a sort of back door: Instead of working within PBS, I could work for one of the outfits that contracted with the station. I wrote, produced, and directed several of my own segments and now had a reel to show of my own work. That gave me the clout to move to other outlets with higher-level production credits.

I almost died when I got hired to work as a postproduction supervisor with Errol Morris, a documentary filmmaker I revered. Errol is a god in the documentary world—one of the few to have had theatrical releases of his films back then. His new show, *First Person*, consisted of in-depth character sketches of individuals in the clutches of deep obsessions: one man was consumed by his passion to capture a living giant squid on camera; another was a fervent pen pal of Ted Kaczynski. This was a fun, gripping gig, and it was by far my most prestigious yet. I was jetting off to New York for sound mixing, or working on color correction and titles with the talented editors. I ate it up, juggling a million tasks to get the show ready for air.

My favorite editor was a dry-witted New Yorker named Doug. He seemed like such a sophisticated, cool guy—funny and sarcastic and very, very talented. Somehow, different as we were, we hit it off big time. Hanging out with Doug made even the longest, most stressful work nights a pleasure. This wasn't a romance; we were both involved with other people. But that didn't stop me from thinking to myself sometimes what life would be like with Doug. He was so laid-back and thoughtful—and I loved watching him work.

During those first couple of years in Boston, I could see that Boogie was losing weight. She was in her late teens and was showing her age. She was no longer the fat kitty with the tiny head that she had always been, and she slept most of the day and night. I could look into her eyes and feel her slowly fading away.

Finally, one night when I came home from work, I could tell that something was wrong. She showed no interest in her breakfast that day, and she wasn't hungry for dinner. I made a vet appointment, dreading the date for fear they'd give me news I couldn't handle. I began to spend long evenings with her cuddled in my lap. I stroked her and spoke to her, hiding the dread in my heart. Sure enough, the vet confirmed that her kidneys were beginning to shut down. There wasn't much that could be done about that for a cat Boogie's age. I began to take her to the vet weekly to check her kidney function, and I gave her IV fluids every night, which made both her and me miserable. I would hold her in my lap and poke a needle in the thin scruff of her neck and speak to her as the fluids dripped in, hoping that she could communicate with me, somehow, after all these years together.

"Please, give me a sign and tell me if you want to continue with this or end it. I'm sorry for the pain I'm causing you—I just want to help. I wish you could tell me. . . ." In the meantime, I did all I could to cherish the moments I had with my sweet friend.

A month into her treatments, Boogie's kidney test showed that they were barely functioning and all the fluids in the world weren't making them work better. To keep her around for myself wasn't the right thing to do.

Boogie and I went to the park one last time. Lying on our blanket in the sun, I snuggled up with her and told her what she'd meant to me all these years. It was painful to know that she was embarking on a series of lasts: last trip to the park, last cuddle, last dinner. She'd been my constant companion, my dear friend, through such enormous and formative swaths of my life, and it seemed impossible that she would no longer be there.

Andy loved her dearly, too, which gave me comfort through the whole ordeal. We took her to a local veterinary hospital and bawled our way through our good-byes. This was my first experience losing an animal friend, and though there have been too many since then, my memory of that moment is still as painful as it is vivid.

Going back to our Allston apartment without Boogie was awful. Everywhere I looked seemed to have a memory of her—the chair where she liked to curl up, the water dish, still half full, the counter she'd jump onto no matter how many times I asked her not to.

Without Boogie there and with the tension between us that had begun to fill our tiny apartment, we both thought a change would be healing. We moved to a groovy loft right on the water in South Boston, a converted distillery that had become a dedicated artist space. This was the first move I'd made without Boogie since I was an adolescent, and there was a space in the van that put a pit in my stomach. But in all other ways, I felt hopeful about this move. We were trying to make a fresh start, and our loft was amazing. The high ceilings, exposed brick, and windows overlooking the bay, the artsy and sociable neighbors—this was the hippest community and apartment I had lived in, and I loved it.

Shortly after the move, I discovered Farm Sanctuary, the first haven for abused, neglected, and discarded farm animals in the country. Somehow, I'd ended up on their mailing list, and the brochure they sent me about their upstate New York pastures was as influential as the ones I'd picked up during college orientation week. I had no idea there was a place dedicated to rescuing farm animals and educating people about farm animal issues. Here was a sanctuary that was actually full of *happy* animals, lucky ones who'd escaped the horrors. I was intrigued. I'd find myself driving along the Charles River, staring at the Boston skyline, dreaming of a visit, and picture myself hugging cows, pigs, and any other animal I could get my hands on.

The books and magazines I began reading were no longer about film production; they were about animals and our use of them. Perhaps the most compelling book I read at that time was Carol Adams's *The Sexual Politics of Meat*, which makes the connection between violence against animals and violence against women.

Adams points out that the most patriarchal societies are also the most carnivorous, and that vegetarianism and feminism are linked. She helped me see a bigger picture of the movement I was becoming a part of, and introduced me to animal rights philosophy and theory. And as someone whose value system had her fighting both sexism and speciesism, I was deeply moved and influenced by Adams's points.

But no matter what book was on my nightstand or what I dreamed about on my commute, I spent most of my time moving my career forward. After a season at *First Person*, I went back to WGBH for a coveted staff position as a postproduction supervisor on the popular documentary series *Frontline*. While that might sound exciting, the job involved a lot of, say, discussing minute details of credits and title placement ad nauseam and sitting in a pitch-black room with glowing monitors for most of the day. It became maddening even though I really liked my colleagues, many there to this day. So after about a year, I left the coveted, benefits-conferring position for one that would bring me out of that dark room and into the field.

Ahhh—freelancing again! I produced a documentary about one man's journey up the Limpopo River in South Africa and a pilot for PBS. Then I landed the crown jewel of my production career: I coproduced and directed a documentary for Discovery Channel's *Extreme Engineering* with my good friend and former coworker Olympia Stone. It was called *The Transatlantic Tunnel*, and it was an enormous and stressful job. We were in charge of writing the

script from a concept, locating and booking crews and equipment overseas, setting up interviews, and on and on. We flew
everywhere—filming fjords in Norway, magnetically levitated
trains in Germany, and tunnel interiors in the Netherlands. I'd
board a transcontinental flight and think about my childhood days
hardly venturing beyond the Ohio River. It was fun and it was
adventurous—but in the end, it wasn't as soul-satisfying as I hoped
it would be. And God, was it stressful—especially since I came
down with a terrible cold during all the traveling and Olympia and
I sometimes wanted to kill each other.

When I came home from a trip, I'd sometimes still look for
Boogie as I set down the suitcase. People kept telling me it
would get easier, but a year after her death I still felt her loss
deeply. That kind of pain is the price we pay for loving. The more
lives we gather into ours, the more loss we're left to deal with. I am
glad to be someone willing to make loss part of my life, since it is
part and parcel of the quality of those rescued lives, but it is endlessly hard.

I made a shrine to Boogie in a Mexican tin *nicho* that I keep in
my office at the sanctuary. It is still a comfort more than a decade
after losing her. There's a tuft of her orange-black-and-white hair, a
little lace pouch containing her ashes, a pen-and-ink illustration of
her that a tattoo-artist friend made for me that reads "Boogie Forever," and photos spanning her life pasted to the *nicho*'s walls.
From my desk in my eclectically decorated (so I like to decorate!)
Mission Control, where cats sun themselves in the window, Coco
the blind chicken runs around squawking, and dogs snore at my

feet, I can see animals grazing in the sheep and goat pastures, free-roaming turkeys, pigs lying in the muddy, shallow pond, the shining disc of the duck pond, and, off in the distance, the swish of Dylan's tail. I often look from that view to her shrine. "Look what we made, Boogie," I tell her.

....

6

Dougable

Quincy the duck was just a tiny yellow ball of fluff when she was abandoned in a park in New York City. Judging by the time of year, we figured she'd been an Easter gift. Parents sometimes think it's a good idea to buy live baby animals to give their children during the holiday. Some ducks and chicks even come dyed in Easter colors: The hatcheries inject a food coloring into the eggshells before they hatch, resulting in perfectly pink, blue, and green little fluffy "toys." And sadly, pet stores enable that by placing irresistible ducklings, chicks, and baby bunnies in the windows for all to see. They are the quintessential icons of the holiday, like the basket decorations and holiday candy. And in New York City, you can have anything you want! Including live animals as gifts.

All too often, the ducklings, chicks, and bunnies that are cherished on Easter day end up getting dropped, stepped on, or otherwise injured—or they are abandoned when the reality of their ongoing care sets in. It's a strange exercise in living in the present and ignoring even the most basic realities of biology. Fuzzy chicks are tiny, sensitive babies who inevitably become full-grown hens and roosters. Ducklings and ducks need water and shelter, and bunnies shouldn't spend the rest of their lives in a small wire cage—although this is typically their plight.

As these realities dawn, people often dump these confused, ill-prepared, and frightened creatures in a parking lot, city playground, or, if they're "responsible," a shelter. Not only is this a trauma for the animal and a headache for the municipality, it doesn't serve a child well to see that kind of behavior as a model. Parents are teaching kids that when they make a bad decision, they can dump it off on someone else and forget about it. Bringing home these Easter "pets" also sends the message that animals are here for our enjoyment and whim, that they are mere trinkets or toys, not feeling individuals. This drives me nuts.

It's difficult to tell the sex of ducklings, so we wanted a gender-neutral name for our new little friend. Dawn Ladd, a dear friend and long-time board member, drove her up from the city and came up with the name Quincy. From the moment she arrived, Quincy couldn't stand to be by herself. As soon as someone put her down, she'd quack at the top of her tiny lungs. Only when we nestled her under our arms and carried her around was she content. It was plain to see that she needed and desired the comfort of a mother's love; it's as instinctual to a duckling as it is to a child to want to feel protected and nurtured. Think of a pond in the springtime, how ducklings cluster behind their mother, all swimming together. And if that mama and siblings aren't around, whoever shows a baby affection and attention is often a good substitute. This isn't true only of ducks, of course; many species will seek out or accept surrogate mothering.

Dougable

A group of us on the farm—including caretakers Rebecca, Julie, Amber, and Phil and a beloved volunteer, Jean Rhode—were now "Quincy's Many Moms," as we called ourselves. She wanted to follow us everywhere we went, but that wasn't feasible. Oh, but hearing her high-pitched quacks at moments of separation was heartbreaking! Luckily, ingenious animal-contraption inventor Rebecca came up with a solution. She found a wine-colored fabric remnant and made an adjustable body sling for the Moms to wear, a sort of BabyBjörn-gone-duck. It kept Quincy close to beating hearts and warm company. Rebecca and other Moms took turns carrying the little duck around in her sling between naps and meals, and all parties were perfectly content.

We'd been talking about developing a duck habitat with a pond before we got the call from city workers about Quincy, but that plan hadn't gotten beyond the idea stage because, as can be expected in the world of nonprofit organizations, we didn't have the funding. So in the meantime, this baby's duck pond would be a kiddie pool. When it came time for her first dip, we all gathered around the little plastic pond to watch and support Quincy. She was adorable, a flash of yellow and orange against the bright blue pool. But when we placed her gently in the water, she was frantic. We could barely keep ourselves from snatching her back out. We knew she wouldn't drown in there and could easily flop herself over the side to rest on the grass, which is exactly what she did the first few times we put her in.

Before long, we could tell that she was starting to enjoy it—her tiny wing nubs flapped like crazy as she motored around. Then she started in on a plunge routine: She'd dunk herself all the way under the water and then emerge just long enough to give herself a good shake, droplets flying, before diving down again. It was insanely cute. We melted into piles of goo. Cartoon bluebirds sang and rainbows were painted on the sky.

Just a few weeks later, Quincy fully comfortable in her new digs (though still following us around quacking), we got a call that another duckling had been found abandoned in a box near the FDR Drive in Manhattan, most likely another Easter casualty. Teddy—he was old enough to have developed a drake feather, so we could tell he was a boy—soon arrived. He was a Pekin duck, like Quincy, the kind usually seen in a Chinese restaurant window plucked and roasted head and all. As always, it felt great to be able to help him avoid that future or a future in a Manhattan bathtub—or getting hit and killed on the FDR! Who would leave him there?!

After we checked Teddy out for parasites and disease and gave him a clean bill of health (pun intended), we couldn't wait to introduce him to Quincy. We were excited for these two little loners to meet and hopefully bond. We set Teddy down on the grass outside the chain-link fence surrounding Quincy's pen. A couple of feet away, Quincy was sunning herself and nudging her wing nubs with her bill. At first, there wasn't much to this fledgling relationship; in fact, they seemed freaked out. They didn't even want to make eye contact. When we tried to put them in the pen together, Teddy would stand at the gate and quack to be let out. Quincy and Teddy may have been with other ducklings for only the first few days of their lives, so they may have forgotten or never developed a bond with them. But we were eager to keep these two together, both because we knew they'd benefit from it and because we had only one duck pen with a swimming pool set up. So we pushed the issue, holding them near each other on opposite sides of the fence a few times a day, a few minutes at a time.

We figured they'd get used to each other eventually, and they did. When we could see they were moving closer to each other without alarm, we moved Teddy into Quincy's pen. There were no more freak-outs; they coexisted, but only just. There still wasn't eye contact. And when one would get in the pool, the other would get out. They were cautiously keeping their distance.

Slowly, over the course of a couple of weeks, as I'd walk over to say hello, I could see that they were sitting a little closer together or were both in the kiddie pool at the same time. Then one day, I caught Teddy preening Quincy, nuzzling her neck with his bill. She returned the favor, digging gently under his wing feathers. Pretty soon, Quincy was so enamored of Teddy that she stopped craving human attention; she was getting all she needed right there in the duck pen. As much as we loved to see that and knew it was best for her, it made us all just a little sad to put away the duck sling for good. Quincy was the bird, but her "Many Moms" were the ones feeling the empty nest.

What a joy it was, though, to marvel at the two of them as their infatuation blossomed. Now they are absolutely inseparable. They talk to each other, groom each other, eat, swim, and sleep together, a real couple. Teddy is fiercely defensive of Quincy. As soon as people come into their area, he quickly waddles over, quacking away, and nibbles their legs as if to say, "She's mine! Get outta here!" He'll follow you wherever you go to make sure you don't get too close to his lady, and he's been known to grab and toss away camera phones and untie shoelaces with disdain when visitors cross the line.

The Lucky Ones

We're a long way from the kiddie pool days: We've now built a beautiful duck and goose habitat with a fountain-fed pond and have introduced many other rescued birds to the sweethearts. They're now friends with Mickey and Jo, who were rescued from the gruesome foie gras industry (think overcrowded sheds, daily force feedings with a tube jammed down the birds' throats, liver disease, and slaughter). And they swim alongside geese Prema and Denise, who, until coming to us, had spent their whole lives, ten *years*, on an "organic" meat and dairy farm with *no access to water* for bathing and swimming—a goose's definition of hell since swimming is what they want to do with every cell of their being. And if that wasn't bad enough, they were living crammed into an overcrowded, filthy shed with four or five hundred hens used for egg laying.

Everyone here has a story.

■ ■ ■ ■

Two years into my time in Boston, Andy and I decided to call it quits. We found ourselves fighting more than loving, which we agreed was no way to live. Now with Boogie and Andy gone, I was on my own again. But I kept the loft and never had a chance to feel lonely, thanks to the incredible cast of characters that were my neighbors in the Distillery. The wild, impromptu dinner parties, open-studio events, late-night knocks at the door from friends who just wanted to stop by—it was never-ending, but it was one of the best times of my life.

Dougable

....

I remember telling my *First Person* colleague Doug about my artificial leg as we sat in the editing room late one night, working on Errol Morris's interview with Clyde Roper, the giant squid seeker. Doug couldn't have given two hoots. For him, it was a non-issue; not titillating or grotesque, just a fact of my life. Maybe he said something blasé like "Oh, that's cool—wow, I wouldn't have known," then continued the previous conversation.

Doug and I had a great working relationship and quickly became friends. I was Errol's postproduction supervisor, and Doug was one of three editors on the show. I was awed by his talent—he had an impressive résumé, full of shows like *Strangers with Candy*, *The Awful Truth* (with Michael Moore), and a film I had seen called *Six Ways to Sunday*. Not to mention the HBO documentary films and other Comedy Central shows. Everyone admired the hell out of him—but I was also charmed by the fact that he was so modest, almost embarrassed, when praised. And he was just such a cool, funny guy. We could all see that Errol had a great deal of respect for him. A great director knows that his most important allies are the cinematographer and the editor, and it is often the editor who carves out the story and creates the captivating scenes. It requires true artistry, especially in the case of documentaries, for which editors have to whittle hundreds of hours of footage into a feature-length film.

But Doug is egoless. And that combined with good looks, insane talent, and the nicest-guy-you'll-ever-meet syndrome—well, I found myself more than a little attracted to him. I loved his goofiness—like the alarm sound he made whenever something embarrassing happened—and his ridiculously dry sense of humor. He'd let go a joke so quickly and so deadpan that you'd almost miss it. He would also go out of his way to be gentlemanly with me, like offering to get me a cup of coffee or making sure I had a comfortable chair while we were screening footage. (I should have been offering these to him, and did, but his time was more precious—and costly—than mine, and he would jump up and be out at the door so quickly that I didn't have time to stop him.) Then there was the pure chemistry between us. We'd often work side by side, staring at a wall of monitors in the online edit or color correction sessions, and if his knee so much as brushed against me, I'd get crazy butterflies in my belly.

But I tried to not allow myself to fantasize about a relationship with Doug. For one thing, I wasn't ready to jump into something—it was too soon after Andy. For another, Doug had been with his girlfriend for five years. I felt more than a little jealous of the mystery woman but didn't see myself as a relationship wrecker.

With the end of the series season coming up quickly, I wondered whether we'd even be able to stay friends. In the TV business, you never know whether a renewal contract was coming or not, and there was a good chance we would never work together again. Besides, I knew Doug was planning to head back to his native Manhattan where he already had another editing gig lined up with *TV Funhouse* on Comedy Central.

It happened that his move back to New York coincided with a trip I was making, so I offered to drive him down. I knew that I was chauffeuring someone I had feelings for right to his girlfriend's door, but I thought we'd have fun on the trip, perhaps our last chance to spend time together.

At first, we talked about the show, Boston, New York, and all the happenings of the past six months we'd worked together, including my leaving Andy. We drove and talked, and sometime during the trip his girlfriend's name came up. He began acting a little strange and reluctantly talked about their plans for the evening. But then he interrupted himself and blurted out something rather mysterious: "She's going to know."

"Know what?" I asked.

He paused, staring straight out at the road, then took a breath and looked over at me. "That I have a huge crush on you."

I felt my jaw drop and my stomach go rigid. A crush? It sounded so high school, yet so endearing. I was dumbfounded. It was the first I knew of the depth of his feelings—or that he truly had any to begin with. He told me he needed to know before walking through that door whether I had feelings for him, too—it was a now-or-never moment, and the answer was clear, though scary to say. I told him, "I do."

The rest of that conversation was a tumble of conflicting thoughts and words. I was nervous about jumping into something too soon, and I was afraid I'd hurt him if I realized I wasn't ready. And I valued Doug so much as a friend, I was terrified of losing him. For his part, Doug said he had a pit in his stomach after admitting his feelings to me. He had been afraid that my feelings weren't reciprocal and now dreaded the prospect of ending a relationship that wasn't broken but had run its course.

"What are we going to do?" I said.

"I'm going to have to tell her," he replied, "but I need some time to figure out how."

When he got out of the car, we hugged in a way we hadn't before; it was an awkward but passionate, scared, we're-not-ready-to-kiss-yet hug. An hour before, I hadn't been sure I'd ever see Doug again, and now we were holding each other. I was reeling. We, of course, decided that it was best that I didn't come up to his apartment, where she would soon be meeting him, as we had originally planned.

I got back into the car. Had I imagined what'd just happened? I drove straight over to see my friends Cesar and Randy and couldn't talk about anything else. But they were hesitant. "Don't get ahead of yourself here," Cesar said. "This is the rebound guy." But I didn't want to think about that. I didn't want it to be true, and I didn't think it was—I'd fallen in love with a friend, which was a stronger foundation to build from than I had ever had before.

Doug called me the next morning and asked to meet later that day at Cedar Tavern, an old bar he knew from his days spending a lot of time at filmmaker Barbara Kopple's nearby studio. I arrived first and sat at a table toward the back, looking over at the door every few seconds. My heart lurched when he walked in and sat down. We talked for hours over a shared bottle of wine, reflecting on our months spent together working and what we were both feeling.

"I got so nervous around you sometimes," he said.

"Me, too!" I smiled.

"Sometimes I'd inch closer to you when we screened footage from the couch," he admitted.

"I always wondered whether you were doing that on purpose,

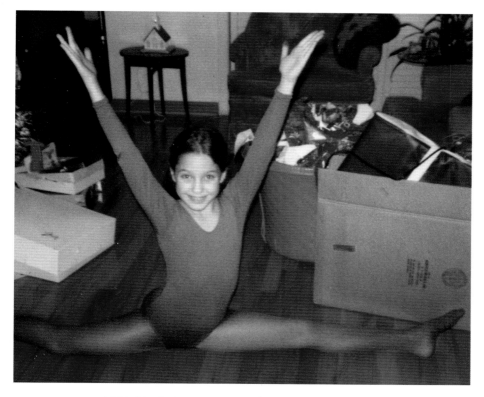

1978 The little gymnast: several years before cancer.

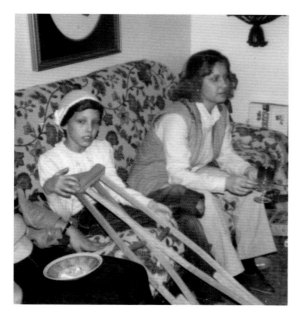

1980

First Christmas post-amputation: undergoing chemotherapy and wearing a wig to hide my bald head.

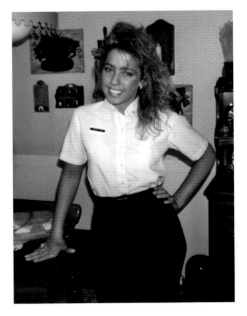

1986

Sweet sixteen, headed to my job at McDonald's (I know . . . that is some terrifying hair!)

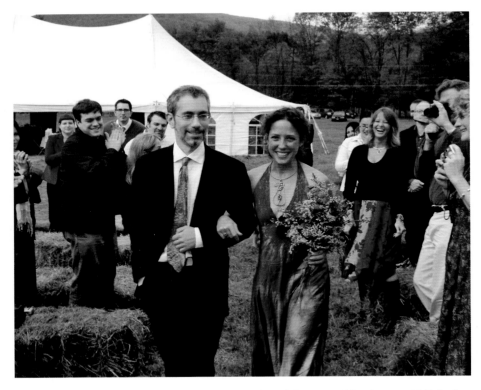

2004 Just months after we bought the Woodstock house and land, we got hitched. Our wedding was the first fund-raiser for the fledgling sanctuary. *(Derek Goodwin)*

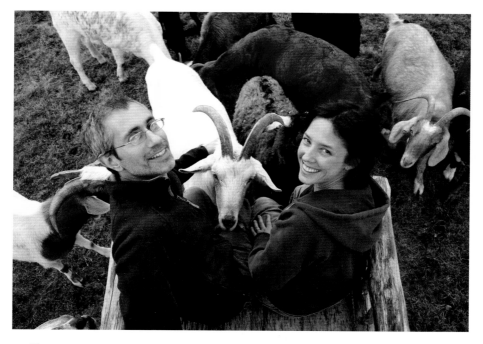

The same pasture where we were married was filled with goats three years later; with Doug, Victor (center), and other friends. *(Derek Goodwin)*

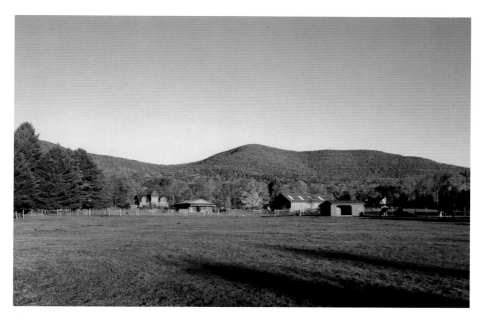

Woodstock Farm Animal Sanctuary in 2007: besides the house, none of these buildings or fences were here when we bought the property in 2004. *(Bob Esposito)*

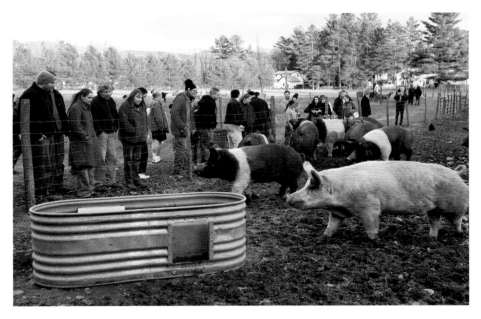

Visitors enjoy watching the pigs get ready for dinner. *(Derek Goodwin)*

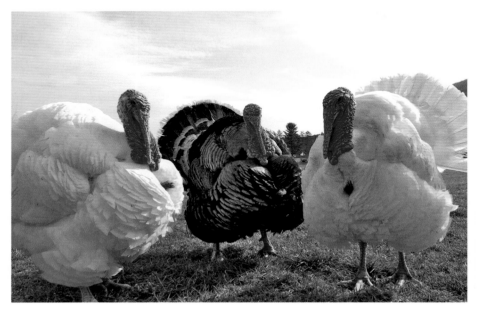

The three wise men: Alphonso, Herschel, and Boone. *(Bob Esposito)*

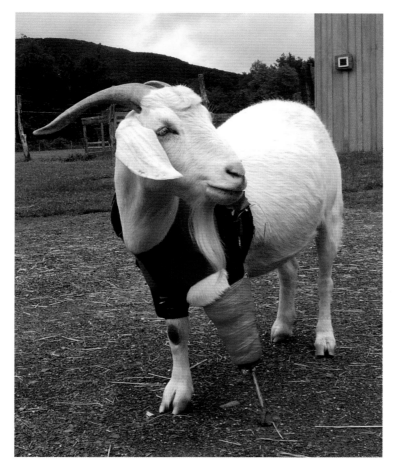

2011 Albie with his prosthetic leg.

2007

Albie when he arrived; our first caregiver, Robin Henderson, and I are treating his maggot-infested leg.

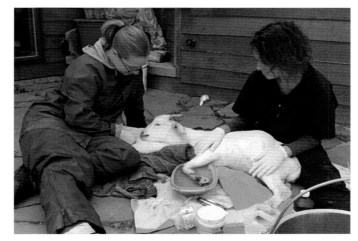

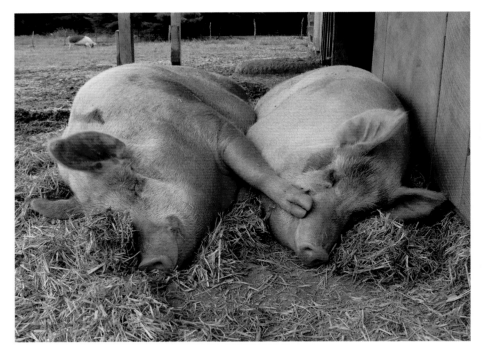

Judy and Patsy, close sisters, enjoy a snuggle.

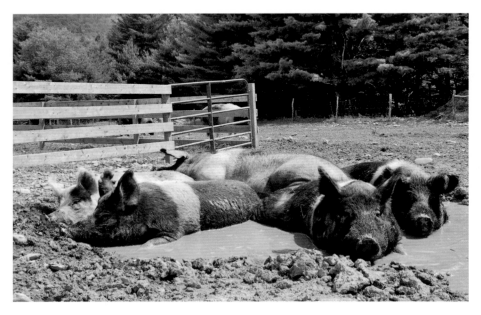

On a hot August day a communal bath is lovely. *(Bob Esposito)*

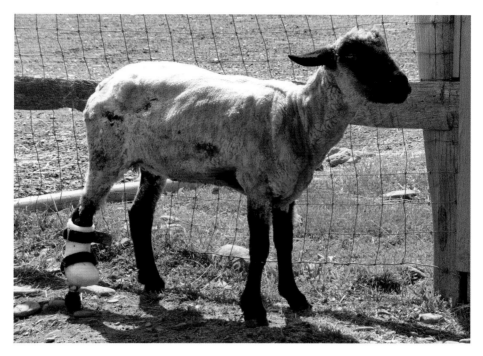

Louise with her corrective brace.

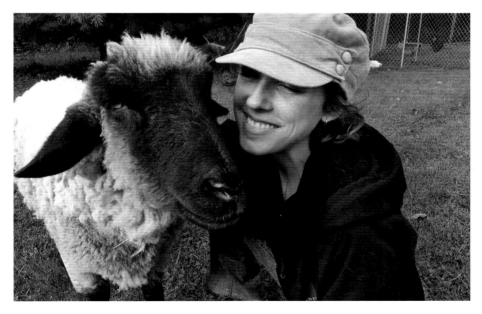

Louise craves human attention, and I love to give it to her as often as I can.
In fact, I crave *her* attention!

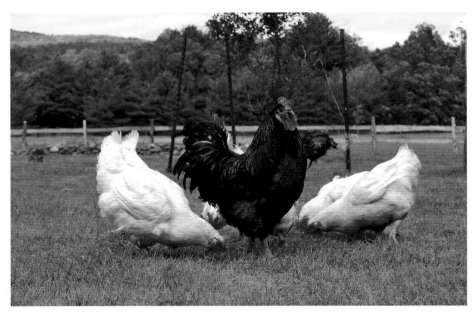

Brandy the rooster stands watch over his hen friends. *(Bob Esposito)*

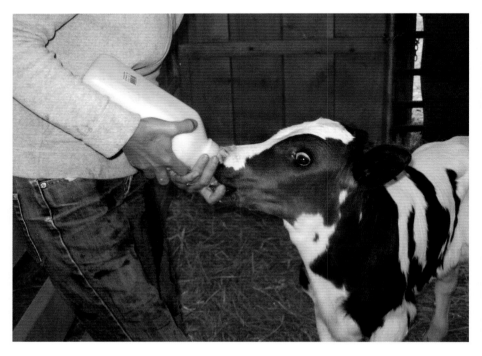

Me feeding Dylan his first meal at the sanctuary.

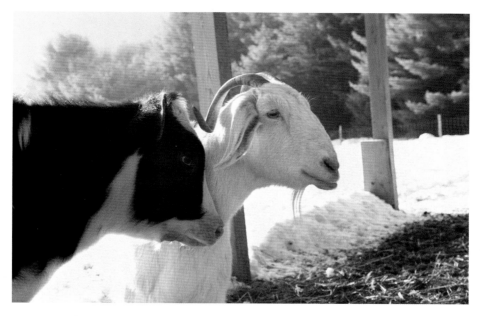

Dylan followed surrogate mom Olivia everywhere. *(Bob Esposito)*

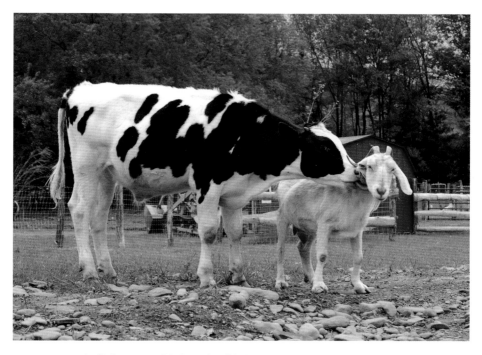

As Dylan grew, his love for Olivia was steadfast. *(Bob Esposito)*

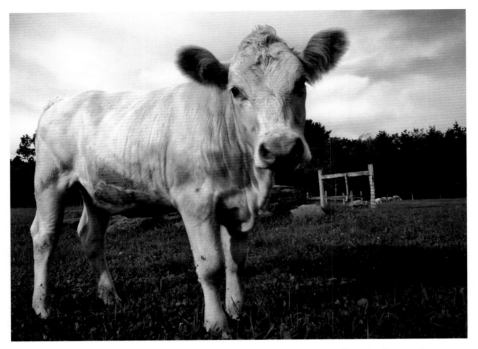

Kayli, a slaughterhouse escapee who received a "pardon" from the governor of Pennsylvania. *(Derek Goodwin)*

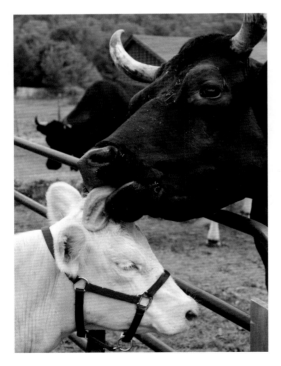

Kayli got some bovine TLC when she first met Andy, a grown-up rescued veal calf.

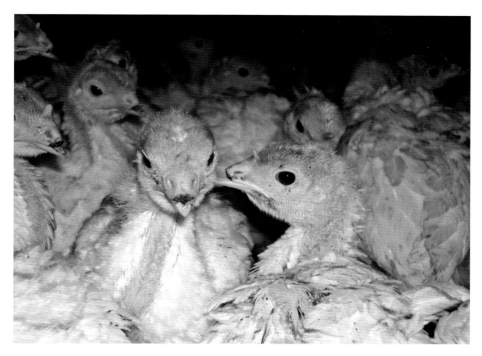

Baby turkeys are painfully debeaked and raised in crowded pens.
(Courtesy Farm Sanctuary, Inc.)

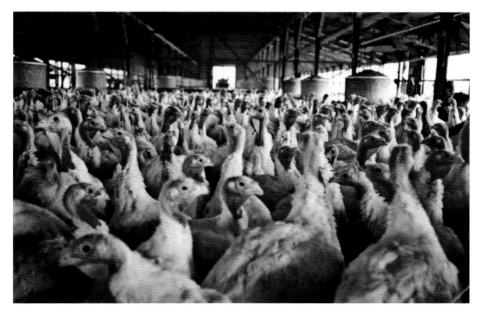

Crowded turkeys in a factory farm.
(Courtesy Farm Sanctuary, Inc.)

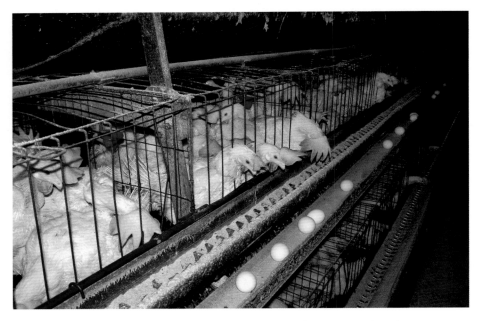

Over ninety-five percent of eggs in the United States come from hens
living their adult lives like this. *(Courtesy Farm Sanctuary, Inc.)*

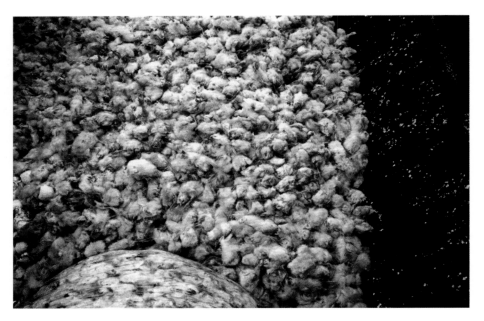

The male chicks of the egg-laying breeds are discarded, or ground up alive.
Only hens are deemed valuable. *(Courtesy Farm Sanctuary, Inc.)*

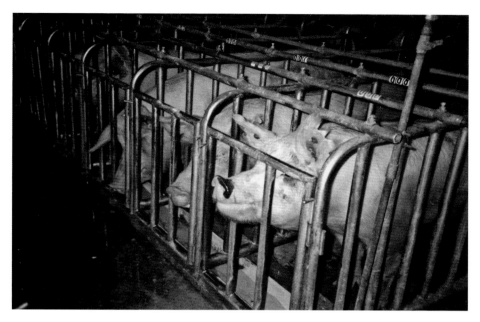

Breeding sows live a life of confinement in twenty-four-inch-wide gestation crates, where they are unable to turn around or even lie down comfortably.
(Courtesy Farm Sanctuary, Inc.)

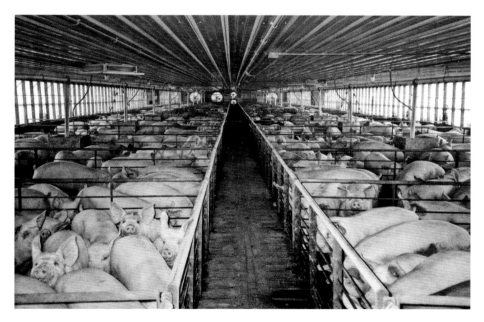

Young pigs are raised in cramped pens until fattened—they are slaughtered after just six months at about 250 pounds. *(Courtesy Farm Sanctuary, Inc.)*

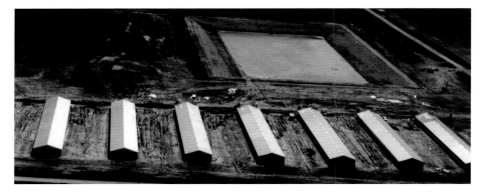

A factory farm for thousands of pigs; note the manure lagoon.
(Courtesy Iowa Citizens for Community Improvement)

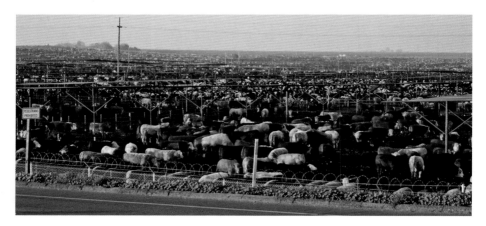

Approximately 35 million cattle are raised for beef each year in the United States. Most are castrated, dehorned, and branded—painful procedures performed without any anesthesia. After grazing on the range for seven months, they are transported to feedlots like the one shown above, where they are fattened on unnatural diets until they reach slaughter weight. *(Courtesy Farm Sanctuary, Inc.)*

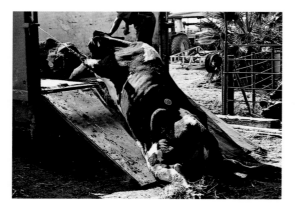

"Downers," animals too injured or weak to walk, are often dragged onto slaughter-bound trucks with tractors and chains.

(Courtesy Farm Sanctuary, Inc.)

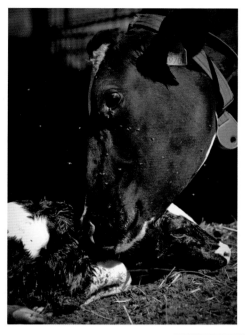

A dairy calf is taken from
her mother still wet from birth,
never to see her again.
(Jo-Anne McArthur)

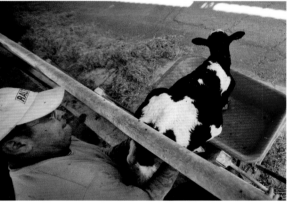

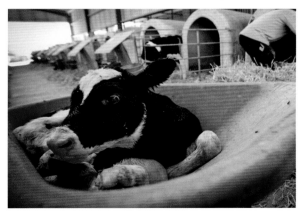

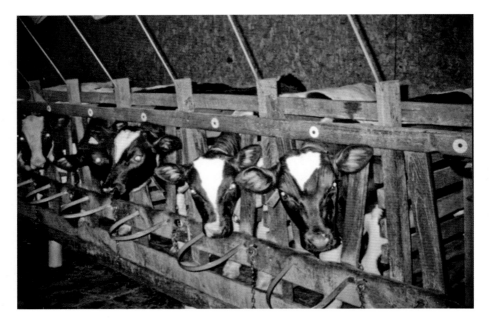

Male calves—"by-products" of the dairy industry—are generally taken from their mothers when they are less than one day old. The calves are then placed in dark, tiny crates, where they are kept almost completely immobilized so that their flesh stays tender. *(Courtesy Farm Sanctuary, Inc.)*

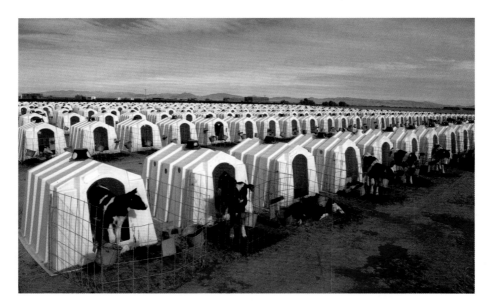

The female calves of dairy breeds, called "replacement calves," are raised in fiberglass huts and artificially inseminated at just fourteen months of age to begin lactation. *(AP/Joe Cavaretta)*

but then I'd do it right back. Colleagues don't usually sit that close, do they?" I laughed.

Then, in one breathless moment, we stopped talking and looked at each other. Our first kiss was magic. Instead of butterflies, I felt like I had roman candles in my belly. But then we talked about his girlfriend and what he planned to do. He dreaded it, but he knew it would feel worse the longer he waited.

Somehow we managed to part ways on the street an hour later. And somehow the next morning, I got back in my car and headed toward home. Once there, my loft felt emptier than ever. It helped that Doug and I talked every day, and that in those pre-9/11 days, you could fly round-trip Boston–New York for less than the cost of a train ticket. We were together every weekend that work allowed and always had a blast, whether we were on a camping trip, at a museum or park, or enjoying a romantic weekend on Block Island or elsewhere in New England.

Then we learned that *First Person* had been picked up for another year, meaning that Doug would be coming back to Boston. Though I wouldn't be working on the show—I'd been hired by *Frontline* in the interim—I knew this meant we could give our relationship a real chance. Doug moved right into my loft. It didn't take long once we were in the same city and the same apartment to see that this was going to be The Relationship for both of us. The hesitancy faded, and the excitement of getting to know each other in a new way took over.

There was only one wrinkle. Doug was no vegetarian. On an early date, as we sat in an Indian restaurant, he ordered lamb. I fought back the urge to say something, but in the end I had to— I just couldn't help myself (but I did wait until after the meal). By then, I'd realized that being preachy on the subject was the surest way to turn people off, so I just asked him if he would mind not ordering such things around me because it was upsetting. I don't tell many people that when I'm out with them, but I knew Doug and felt it was important to let him know. He apologized, and I was happy with his sincere response. He also said that he always found meat kind of icky and he never liked to cook it. In fact, most of his meals were vegetarian, for health and gross-out reasons, but he'd never stopped to really think about the animals, about why we eat animals and whether we should.

The thing was, Doug knew how to ask questions. He was the kind of person who was open to rethinking habits, personally and socially. Over the course of that first summer together, he made it clear that he wanted to know about vegetarianism and the cruelty that farm animals are subjected to on large and small farms alike. I told him things I'd learned from organizations, research, and friends, and he read the newsletters that came to the house from Farm Sanctuary, PETA, and other organizations. I was so happy and relieved to see how affected he was by what he was learning.

Doug started ordering vegetarian food in restaurants, and he stocked the fridge with more produce, grains, and meat alternatives. We tried new recipes together out of vegetarian cookbooks that were usually *off the charts*. Within weeks, meat disappeared from his diet completely. His new way of thinking and eating were cemented when we went to Farm Sanctuary together for a weekend and spent time with rescued farm animals. When he met the sweet sheep and knelt down to scratch them while eye-to-eye, he thought about eating lamb and the thought repulsed and shamed him. He was making the connection. This while I went about the barn in my hugging frenzy.

Although I didn't fall in love with a vegetarian, I fell in love with an open-minded, kindhearted person who was as affected as I had been when I first took a good look at what farm animals endure in their shortened lives. I think I loved and admired Doug more because I got to watch him go through his metamorphoses. We were from radically different backgrounds, New York Jew versus Southern Baptist Belle, but when it came to eating meat, both of those backgrounds included lots of it—without a lot of questioning. Our ethics, values, and outlook of the world were becoming simpatico.

7

Texas, Undercover

He leapt from the truck, weaved through traffic, and bolted down Fifth Avenue in Bay Ridge, Brooklyn, chased the whole way. This was no fugitive or robber: it was Herbie, a frightened Hereford calf.

Herbie, at just four months of age, saw an opportunity to escape his unfortunate fate when his owner and transporter tried to move him from one truck to another at a busy intersection. Herbie made a break for it, slipping his rope and running down the street. With his handler and soon several cops in hot pursuit, Herbie caused traffic jams and stunned pedestrians throughout the neighborhood. Finally, authorities managed to tranquilize and capture him.

According to our laws and societal norms, Herbie was nothing but a piece of property and as such was going to be returned to his owner and his destiny as dinner. But, miraculously, the owner couldn't find the appropriate paperwork to show proof of "ownership," so the police confiscated Herbie and contacted the borough's Center for Animal Care and Control (CACC) instead. The shelter may have housed the occasional ferret or chickens among the many cats and dogs, but it'd sure never taken charge of a calf. This was news! When the local CBS channel aired the story, there was an immediate, passionate outcry to save Herbie.

There is an interesting psychological phenomenon when the media covers a slaughterhouse fugitive. That story has the ability to affect people in a way that a herd headed to slaughter, a hundred Herbies, doesn't. It's easier for people to see animals as individuals when one breaks from the crowd and tries to run for his or her life: "I guess that one really wanted to live!" they think. But of course the ones who are unable to run are no less deserving or desiring of freedom. The opportunity to escape may not present itself, or animals may be too ill to muster the strength to break free, but that does not mean they don't want to be spared. As the Buddha said, "All beings tremble before violence. All fear death, all love life. See yourself in others. Then whom can you hurt? What harm can you do?"

I think it's easier, too, for us to identify with a single animal's plight more than with the millions around them, because the sheer numbers are overwhelming—10 *billion* land animals are slaughtered for human consumption annually in this country alone. I'm glad that a rogue individual, especially one who has been named, will compel people to protest, but I pray for the day when we see every calf on that truck as a Herbie and cry out for each and every one.

Texas, Undercover

■ ■ ■ ■

When Herbie was finally corralled and settled in at the CACC, Sabrina, one of the center's officers who I'd spoken with before, gave us a call. "What have you got for me, Sabrina?" I asked excitedly.

"You've heard about the calf running around Brooklyn?" she asked.

"How could I not? We must have had ten calls from supporters and others already—but this is the one I've been hoping for."

The news had shown pictures of Herbie behind chain-links in an outdoor dog pen at the shelter, munching some hastily procured hay off the concrete and winning the hearts of every staff member and visitor there. I was eager to see him in a field, grazing happily with other cows, a natural place for a cow to be. Still, it was heart-warming to see people connect to him, people who—like me only a few years before—had never interacted with a (live) cow. My heart reeled when I later heard Sabrina on the news saying, "My family and I eat steak and hamburger all the time—we never even think about it. Now, I don't know if I can anymore." Her interview took place right in front of Herbie's pen, helping to make that important connection to all who saw the segment. And in the final local CBS coverage of the rescue, the reporter, Pablo Guzman, said that he thought people were moved by Herbie's story partially because of the holiday season: "It is that time of year," he said, "when a child born in a manger surrounded by animals reminded us that we are all—people and animals—unique and living creatures bound together." That was beautifully phrased, and Doug and I were thrilled, though I wish such sentiments were expressed in *every* season.

A few hours later, a red VW camper van rumbled its way into our driveway. Behind the wheel was our own Dawn Ladd, and in the back was a tarp to protect the carpeting and a gorgeous brown-and-white calf. It was official: Instead of a slaughterhouse, courageous Herbie had found safe haven and love at the end of his ride. But, poor boy, he didn't look or feel so great when he arrived. He was underweight and dirty, with a numbered sticker on his back, a numbered tag in his ear, and an upset stomach (the diarrhea attested to that, and despite the tarp, Dawn's van was never the same). Herbie was led to the isolation stall in our pig barn—the same one where young Dylan had stayed—and feasted on hay and napped in warm, comfy piles of soft rye straw. He was timid at first, having known only rough handling and unfriendly voices, but within days he allowed himself to enjoy a gentle touch and the company of humans who spoke to him in hushed, sweet tones. What a joy watching him relax into his new life.

I can't talk about Herbie without also mentioning a new slaughterhouse escapee who arrived here at the time of writing this book—the now famous Kayli. Like Herbie, young Kayli was headed for slaughter, this time at a small halal live-kill market just outside Philadelphia. But unlike Herbie, Kayli saw exactly what was going to happen to her. When a worker tried to unload her into the market, she could sense the fear of the other terrified animals crowded into the holding pen. She saw the meat hooks from which hung freshly killed and skinned carcasses. She could smell the blood and fear and death in the room. She fought against her lead hard enough to pull loose and make a mad dash. The workers tried to go after her, but she was far too fast and strong. She ran through the streets, looking for refuge for over an hour before finding herself cornered by police cars. As officers tried to lasso her with dog leashes tied together, Kayli tried again to run, smashing her head into one the car doors in an effort to move the blocked car from her path. But the officers managed to capture her and brought her back to the slaughterhouse.

Marianne Bessey, a local attorney and animal activist, heard about the escaped cow from a neighbor. The news had picked up the story during the chase and even showed a photo of Kayli in the holding pen along with the other doomed animals. Marianne started calling the slaughterhouse, hoping to beg for Kayli's life, but the worker on the other end spoke little English. Marianne felt hopeful enough that she contacted us to see if we could take Kayli in if she won her release. The next morning, though, the workers never showed up. They must have become intimidated by the press and the other activists Marianne had contacted (and some she didn't) who were gathered outside the market. Somehow it came to light that the owner was out of the country, and the workers didn't know how to handle the situation—so they just didn't come in to work.

It was time for a new strategy. Elissa Katz, friend and supporter of WFAS who is also a Philadelphia-based attorney, contacted the Council on American-Islamic Relations, hoping for assistance in mediation. Thanks to the council's director, Moein Khawaja, and a long day of negotiations with both the slaughterhouse owner and state officials, Kayli's freedom was won, if hard won. Pennsylvania law states that an animal must be slaughtered within ten days of arriving at a slaughterhouse unless the market has a special permit to sell live animals (and this one didn't). In fact, in order for the market to stay compliant with the law, Kayli would have to be granted a reprieve by the highest state authority. And miraculously, that's what happened: She was granted an official "pardon" by Pennsylvania Governor Tom Corbett and the state's Department of Agriculture.

What a story and what a happy ending, one I'm reminded of daily when I look out of my office window and watch Kayli graze contentedly—never to end up hanging from a hook. But I'm also reminded that it was only her unique set of circumstances that resulted in her freedom, and all the other animals in that slaughterhouse were not so lucky. That thought is pervasive as I gaze out at all the friends enjoying life here, and it's what gets me going in the morning (along with some strong coffee—I'm an addict!).

In the world of animal welfare, it doesn't take long to stumble across the work of Farm Sanctuary. Back in 1986, Gene Baur and Lorri Bauston started the organization—the first farm animal sanctuary in the United States—when Gene rescued a ewe. While he was filming and investigating a pile of dead animals outside a slaughterhouse, he saw a sheep on top of the pile lift her head: It was Hilda, who had been left for dead because, as it turned out, she was suffering from dehydration. The rehabilitated Hilda became the symbol for the work of Farm Sanctuary and helped launch a paradise for thousands of rescued animals over the years, as well as a cause for thousands of human supporters around the world.

When I learned of Farm Sanctuary, I felt in touch with something noble, something righteous. I couldn't wait to check it out for myself. After supporting the organization and keeping tabs on it from Boston for a year, I received a mailer that publicized Farm Sanctuary's annual Critter Care Conference: a way for people to spend a weekend on site at the sanctuary, in the Finger Lakes region of New York, to see what caring for farm animals and running a sanctuary were all about.

Aside from the occasional childhood petting zoo experience, my only face time with farm animals was at the annual Kentucky State Fair. I loved going to see and pet them in the "livestock" exhibits, but I always left depressed. Seeing the animals lined up and tethered on short leads or in pens with numbered tags in their ears made me stop and question why we have the right to own them and exhibit them this way—like slaves. They bore numbers. Not names.

Manhattanite Doug had grown up with cats and visited the Central Park and Bronx zoos as a child. But farm animals? No . . . nothing.

And both of us were just beginning to really absorb the scope of the abuse of farm animals in the United States alone. Compared with the number of farm animals living and dying each day, dogs and cats are hardly a blip on the screen. Ditto lab, fur, and circus animals. Of course, I would never stop advocating on behalf of those populations, either, but I could hardly get my head around the fact that farm animals make up a staggering ninety-eight percent of domestic animals in this country.

I was beginning to feel the need to refocus my life and engage more in animal advocacy, and I was dying to get up close and personal with *happy* farm animals who would never be killed or used for any reason. I needed the comfort and reassurance that there were good people out there rescuing farmed animals and providing them sanctuary. I wanted to see them and touch them and look into their eyes. I asked Doug to go with me, and being the supportive guy he is, he obliged. I think he thought I was a little meshuga, as his people say.

Even though we were living it up in our urban digs, I daydreamed about buying some property and adopting some cows or perhaps a few pigs and chickens and who knows . . . maybe starting a sanctuary of my own some day. It was a ridiculous pipe dream, of course. I didn't know anything about caring for them, nor was I certain I could pull something like that off. But it certainly couldn't hurt to get to know some real-life farm animals and learn more about their personalities and what it takes to care for them. And I wanted to learn how to effectively advocate on their behalf without having people tune me out. At the time, I was talking a lot more with friends and colleagues about why I was vegetarian, and I would often get the "No, don't tell me . . . I don't want to know" response, which frustrated the hell out of me. Willful ignorance is something I just can't respect, and feeling frustrated, I found that I was distancing myself from them and not having the tools to deal with such situations constructively. Yet I was guilty of some ignorance as well. At this point, we were still eating dairy and eggs, and lots of each. Doug and I had an egg sandwich almost every day, thinking the protein was essential since we didn't eat meat, and we reveled in all sorts of cheeses. We would go into a been-there-forever cheese shop near a weekend farmers' market and ask, "What's the stinkiest cheese you have?"

On Critter Care Conference weekend, we started our seven-hour drive in notoriously awful downtown Boston traffic and ended it in western New York, with rolling hills and green everywhere. Large- and small-scale animal farming operations bordered the roads of our journey, as did ads for hunting associations and turkey shoots. We were both struck by an eerie feeling that we were in Alien Territory. We landed in the tiny town of Watkins Glen, grabbed dinner, and checked into our hotel for the night.

The next morning, we headed out of town and down a winding road toward Farm Sanctuary. After almost losing our lunch on a pothole-pocked dirt road, we came out of a bend to find a picturesque farm with expansive fields on a hillside. In the foreground I saw a group of enormous pink pigs hanging out and swimming around in a pond. I turned to Doug and said, "I think we're going to like this place! I can't wait to meet those pigs!!!" We drove up the road to get a better look, then turned around by a small yard of white chickens to head back to our destination. "This place is paradise," I said, squeezing Doug's hand. He was too busy being a fish out of water to react, but his MO often involved making sure I was happy, and that I was. I drove back down the potholed road to the People Barn, the sanctuary's visitors' center. We walked in and saw other conference attendees finding a seat, sipping coffee, and looking at the photos of famous vegetarians and supporters of the organization that covered one wall. Another wall displayed images of animals in various forms of confinement in factory farms and to-scale replicas of the kinds of pens and crates used. My heart sank. Farther down the wall were even sadder images of mutilated animals, animals strung up on the slaughter lines, "downed" animals, and other horrifying images. My eyes welled up as I read a quotation, framed and mounted among the images, from Paul

McCartney: "If slaughterhouses had glass walls, everyone would be a vegetarian."

After a bit of orientation and discussion, we all headed out for the farm tour. This was no Kentucky State Fair. This was a place where we learned of suffering but saw joy; where we saw firsthand the worst and best in humanity. I met turkeys who came up to examine my shiny buttons and enjoy a stroke on the head. I saw cows come running when their names were called and pigs roll over for belly rubs. I'd never experienced anything even a little bit like this. This place, so remote, so embedded in "enemy territory," was a blissful, self-reliant community of good, energetic people caring for animals and working to change hearts and minds.

Ignorance is a funny thing. There's no question that I wish I didn't know some of what I learned that weekend. It was painful to hear a lot of the information, but I knew I'd feel ashamed to turn away now, after what I learned and seeing the scars those animals bore. I reached for my inner Albert Schweitzer, reminding myself to "think occasionally of the suffering of which you spare yourself the sight."

As we headed into one of the many chicken barns, I learned that weekend that the United States kills 14,000 chickens each minute. Fourteen *thousand*. Each *minute*. That's nine billion a year in this country alone—billion with a *b*—50 billion worldwide. It's hard for the human mind to comprehend that volume of death— yet it's somehow possible for humans to carry out.

I learned that a quarter billion baby male chicks—the unwanted by-products of the egg industry—are also killed annually in the country alone. They are ground up alive or suffocated to death in enormous plastic bags thrown into dumpsters.

When we spread out into one of the massive cow pastures, I learned that the United States slaughters millions of dairy cows, who would naturally live twenty to twenty-five years if healthy, at around age four or five. When they head to slaughter, their bodies are so completely wasted after years of overmilking that many of them can't even walk onto the trucks that take them to slaughter. They have to be dragged or forklifted onto the waiting trucks.

I learned that we force pigs into gestation crates and artificially impregnate them, moving them to even narrower crates when they give birth, taking their newborns away after two to three weeks to fatten the babies for slaughter, then starting the cycle over again. They never live outside crates barely bigger than their own bodies, never walk freely or even step outside, and they lose their minds. No one puts it better, perhaps, than Matthew Scully in his book *Dominion*. Scully, erstwhile speechwriter for George W. Bush and a die-hard vegan, pulls no punches about how most farm animals live and just how automated modern-day agriculture has become:

> About 80 million of the 95 million hogs slaughtered each year in America, according to the National Pork Producers Council, are intensively reared in mass-confinement farms, never once in their time on earth feeling soil or sunshine. Genetically designed by machines, inseminated by machines, fed by machines, monitored, herded, electrocuted, stabbed, cleaned, cut, and packaged by machines—themselves treated like machines "from birth to bacon"—these creatures, when eaten, have hardly ever been touched by human hands.

And all of that was just the beginning of what I learned at Farm Sanctuary.

I think the only reason I didn't go jump into nearby Seneca Lake is that I was learning all of this with the understanding that something could be done about it—something *had* to be done about it—and that I could be part of the movement doing something.

Even as I was learning about the horrors, I was being introduced to the other side of things: I was finally meeting chickens, pigs, cows, and others who'd escaped their fates and had learned, for the most part, to trust people again. Many were far friendlier than I had imagined and would approach our group as we entered their barns and pastures. I played with goats, smelling their earthy smells and scratching their coarse fur as we loaded hay into their hay racks. I cuddled chickens, wincing as I saw their seared-off beaks. I pressed my face into Precious the cow's neck, her warmth seeping into my cheek, and sat down with Thelma and Louise, sheep sisters who came right up and nuzzled me for attention. I cleaned Keri the pig's ears for a caretaking assignment and gave her a big belly rub afterward. I never knew pigs could be so talkative and respond to their names when called and that they so thoroughly loved belly rubs and having their ears cleaned. As we spent time with each species, Susie Coston, the shelter director, talked to us in detail about what kind of care is needed: what to feed them, what the medical care is like, what kind of structures and space and bedding they need, how to store their food and supplies, what kind of parasite treatments they need, illnesses they face, what their social dynamics are like. Nothing was sugarcoated—it was hard work caring for hundreds of animals. But damn if she didn't look happy doing it.

Then Susie walked us through one of the banes of animal care: the necessary trimming of pig tusks.

If you learn nothing else from this book, learn this: PIGS HATE TO BE TETHERED. But when one of them is 1,000 pounds to your 125, guess who has to be tethered? Cutting the tusks back doesn't hurt them (no nerve endings in the teeth to the gum), and it has to be done with pigs who otherwise would use them against one another during spats and territorial issues. But the tethering really freaks them out. So Charlie was chosen as the reluctant participant and led into a stall. Susie readied the Gigli wire saw, which I'd never seen, but one that might have been a close match to the one used on my leg during my amputation since that is what it's intended for—it's a surgical bone saw. She donned protective eye wear and stuffed plugs into her ears. I wondered what in the world she needed them for, but as soon as she slipped the rope around Charlie's upper jaw and snout and secured the other end to a wooden post, I knew why. Charlie started up a scream that defined *bloodcurdling*. My veins were suddenly filled with (vegan) cottage cheese. It was a high-pitched, ear-piercing, sustained scream that had all the terror of the world in it. I recognized that what I was hearing was the same cry of every single pig that was being slaughtered at that moment, and had been slaughtered earlier that day, and would be slaughtered that evening, and the next morning, and on and on and on, million upon million—I'd never heard anything like it—it was unbelievably upsetting and unexpected. I burst into tears.

The Lucky Ones

Charlie's terror lasted all of three minutes. The moment the tether was off, he shut up, trotted away, and lay down like nothing had happened. He'd now go back to the bliss of his life, unlike 99.99999999 percent of pigs who scream his scream.

Susie pulled off her gloves, let out a big breath, and caught my eye. She saw my red, snot-covered face, and she said, "Girl, you'd better toughen up if you want to do this!" I laughed and resolved that I'd do just that, but she made fun of me for years.

We stayed in the pig barn awhile. I couldn't get enough of watching Susie in her element, full of expertise and passion and knowledge of these amazing animals. She was explaining other medical procedures and talking about the feeding and maintenance of the pigs. We stepped outside to see some pigs who were bopping around in the sunshine, and I was struck by the sudden appearance of pig turds. Pigs, like dogs, never soil their sleeping areas, and so they do their bathroom business alfresco. So much for the term "filthy pig." "How often do you have to clean up out here?" I asked. "Looks like they poop a lot."

"Oh, yeah," she replied. "We need to scoop in here every day. Whole lot of these around." With that, Susie leaned down to pick up a big old pig turd. Picked it up with her bare hands. I liked Susie from the first minute, but after that I loved her. Watching her stand there tossing that poop like a baseball made me want to be Susie's best friend.

For his part, Doug was plenty moved as well, if a bit horrified by the human-skin-on-pig-poop incident (he made a concerted effort not to shake her hand at the end of the tour). His first love there was the goats. To this day he calls goats "the gateway drug." In their eagerness for affection and connection with humans, they remind us too much of dogs to ignore, yet goats are the most con-sumed "red meat" animals on the planet. And once you've taken that pill, it's easy to see that cows and pigs are also responsive, affectionate, and unique, and then you start noticing the same thing about chickens and turkeys, and then before you know it, you've done gone over to the vegan side.

Both Doug and I understood by day two of the weekend that our dairy days were over. Meeting the dairy cows and egg-laying chick-ens, and meeting the grown-up sons of dairy cows who "should" have become veal years before, made us both realize we never wanted animal products of any kind to pass through our lips again. I loved cheese omelets, but now I was haunted by the image of the critters I'd gotten to know, and I knew I'd feel complicit in the ruth-less treatment of cows and chickens if I consumed their "products." Doug and I made a commitment to go vegan that very day. He may have followed me into vegetarianism, but we were taking this joyful leap into veganism together, and it felt great. "Leap" might be the wrong word to use, since it implies there is a danger involved. How about: We took a step up.

On Sunday, I pulled Farm Sanctuary cofounder Gene Baur aside. "I'd like to offer my skills," I told him. "I'm in film, and it's been about a decade since I went undercover, but I've done it and I have what it takes. I'm willing to go back out on the front lines if you ever have a need."

"I very well may take you up on that, Jenny," he said. "Let me get your information—and, well, thank you!"

I contacted him within a day or so of returning to Boston and relayed my work experience by phone. I told him of the undercover work I had done for PETA and that I was ready to dive back in. A week later, I got a call from him. "What do you know about the Downed Animal Protection Act?" he asked me.

Remember the dairy cows I mentioned who are too sick or injured to walk or even stand when they're brought to slaughter? They are called "downers," and they are by no means the only ones. Because of the abuse and neglect inherent in large-scale farming, *millions* of animals per year—pigs, beef cattle, dairy cows, sheep, calves, and others—are dragged to slaughter with chains, pushed with tractors or forklifts, poked with electric prods, or pulled by their limbs because they cannot physically walk onto the trucks. But no matter how sick or lame they are, companies will not euthanize them because by law animals must be alive when they reach the kill floor if they are to be slaughtered and sold for consumption. It's a horror show.

Gene was working hard to have the U.S. Congress pass the Downed Animal Protection Act, a bill that would mandate humane euthanasia for nonambulatory animals, those who can't stand and walk on their own, and prevent them from being used as food. The subtext is that farmers would then have a financial incentive to treat the animals better and give veterinary attention to the sick. Gene knew we needed people to *see* the suffering of these animals firsthand. That's where I came in. As someone with gumption and filming experience, I could use a hidden camera to document downers at stockyards.

Stockyards are where farmers come to unload their animals for meat packers to buy and take away to slaughter. The animals are auctioned off over the course of a week or so, and then it starts again—one day sheep and goats, the next day dairy cows, and so on. It's a flurry of unloading, buying, selling, trading, and loading up again. Animals are packed into pens, often without food or water for hours or even days, and then herded through the auction ring so bidders from meat-packing companies can get a closer look. For many animals, it's the last stop before the slaughterhouse. Large livestock trailers wait outside to load them up and take them to slaughter.

Gene left the camera research to us film geeks. Back in Boston, Doug and I did our homework and figured out what would work best. Once the palm-size camera arrived in the mail, Doug helped me design a hidden purse device. A hole in the recessed side of the bag let the lens peek out discreetly, and a hole drilled into the plywood base allowed for a tripod bolt. The bolt had a quick-release lever so that if opportunity arose, I could remove the camera quickly for more accurate shooting. I practiced a little in the apartment until I felt confident. The next morning, Doug drove me to the airport, and I was on my way.

No amount of preparation could have lessened the shock of what I encountered in Texas. Almost as soon as I slammed the door of my rental truck at a San Angelo auction, I saw dead, dying, and debilitated animals lying among the living, baking in the hundred-degree heat in pen after pen after pen as far as I could see. Already sweating, I walked over to the first fenced paddock I saw. Right in front of me, many dozens of black-and-white Holsteins, dairy cows, languished there, drooling and panting among dry water troughs. Some had bloody, infected, sore udders, so swollen that the teats were almost dragging the ground. Some were so pregnant that they looked ready to give birth right there in the dust. Because many of the cows' tails had been hacked off, they had no way to swat at the flies that covered their backs and legs. I backed away, turned around to another pen, and saw a huddle of baby Holstein calves slated for veal farms. Their umbilical cords fresh, and some with hides slick with afterbirth, more calves were being dragged out of a truck by their ears, pulled by a leg, or kicked to get up and walk. I could feel tears well up but I fought them back. I couldn't let on where my sympathies lay. A giant sign hung just steps from where I stood: NO PHOTOS OR VIDEO ALLOWED. It was directed at people like me. (You can find an edited version of my footage on YouTube: just search for "Texas stockyards Jenny Brown.")

I closed my eyes for a moment. Breathed in, out. Maybe I could keep a clear head, keep my sanity, if I got to work and started filming. The only way to survive this was to make the experience productive. I found a secluded area, sat down on a set of stairs, and reached into my purse to turn on the hidden camera. While I rummaged, two young men in cowboy hats who'd been dragging and kicking the calves a moment earlier yelled my way. "Hey," they said. I quickly turned on the camera and flicked the viewfinder toward me so that I could see what I was filming. The guys would have no idea what I was doing if I acted fast and kept my cool. "What are you doing?" one of them asked.

I pulled out a notebook. "I guess someone didn't tell you I would be here," I ad-libbed. "I'm a journalist, doing a story about the dairy industry." They looked a little less skeptical. "What about you guys?" I continued. "Do you work here all the time, or are you usually on the farms?"

"Naw, just here, pretty much," one answered. "It's a job." He used his already sweat-soaked T-shirt to wipe his face. I looked over at the animals behind them. A tiny calf, still slick with tongue marks from his mother's grooming, was trying to walk but wasn't quite succeeding. "What about that little guy?" I asked. "He can't seem to walk so well—what's up with him?"

"Oh, he was probably just born this morning."

I blinked and inhaled slowly, careful to mimic their emotionless faces as best I could. I kept them talking long enough for them to get bored of me and head back to work. Then I tried to swallow the lump in my throat.

Once they'd walked away to keep pushing and kicking and pulling calves, I used my discreet spot to set the lens and get going. I picked up my purse and walked over to another filthy holding pen. This one held another group of little male Holsteins, again probably brought in by local dairy farmers to be sold to veal farmers. Some were clumped together in a corner, some unable to stand yet on their brand-new legs. I looked back at the men in the other pen and saw a calf reach up to one of their hands, trying desperately to suckle a dirty finger.

Then I spotted a calf who seemed to have something wrong with his leg and was crying. After a minute, camera rolling, it became clear that he was trying to set weight on a leg that was broken. The calf's limb dangled below the knee, dead and flopping, but the little calf kept trying to put weight on it anyway. What had happened to him? I kept the camera trained on his painful, awkward attempts to maneuver. He may have been trampled, or pulled roughly from his mother's womb. More likely he'd been dragged by that leg, common handling, as I had just witnessed, so roughly that it'd been yanked clear of the joint.

I wanted to climb the fence, gather him into my arms, lay him gently in the backseat of my rental, and drive him to safety. I wanted to deliver him to the most competent veterinarian in the country and then to Susie Coston's arms. I wanted to visit him yearly at Farm Sanctuary, watching him thrive and grow confident and huge. But I couldn't. All I could do was stand there and listen to the workers behind me, joking and laughing as they pulled more calves off the truck. I kept the camera trained on the calf while I repeated under my breath, "I'm so sorry, I'm so sorry, I'm so sorry. . . ."

The ground was opening underneath me.

I had to stop and literally remind myself, again, to breathe and not cry. And on top of it all, I was terrified someone would find me out—would see that I was an enemy because I had a camera and a heart.

I willed my legs to move and walked up the stairs to the metal catwalk used to view animals from above. Underneath me, I saw a group of goats moving through the alleyway toward the building. One had an injured leg and was so pregnant I wondered if she had twins inside. She was being herded toward the auction ring by workers who joked in Spanish while they hit her with a stick that had a plastic bag attached to one end because she was falling behind the others. (I later learned that the sound of the bag scares the animals.) The look of fear on the pregnant goat's face and her effort to walk quickly were enough to make me want to drive a nail through my forehead.

Texas, Undercover

I kept moving with my purse locked to my side, filming all the while. I looked out as far as I could into the pens and saw animals panting, miserable in the heat and desperate for water—why couldn't they at the very least provide them with that? Maybe they had earlier and it was all gone by now, or maybe they didn't care to take the time to do it. It was unbelievable; I saw a cow with blood dripping down her face from a rotting, cancerous eye. Flies and dust covered the wound. Here, too, there was no water in the pen and no shade. Then I saw, languishing in an isolated pen, a huge steer who looked as if he had a broken pelvis. He was foaming at the mouth, covered with flies, but he couldn't get to the puddle of filthy water in the bottom of his trough because he couldn't stand, let alone walk. This was a downer, I suspected, who would lie there neglected until the skid steer came around to drag him or forklift him onto the truck. I wanted so desperately to offer water to him, but I knew I'd be caught. I felt sick. I wanted to scream. I wanted to take each of the workers' heads and bash them into the metal railings. Awful thoughts. And I wondered if I could get to my next destination and have enough time to see the steer loaded onto the truck, but my planned itinerary didn't allow for it.

I walked and filmed, my heart in my throat, my stomach in a twist. I saw a sheep with a prolapsed uterus—most likely from too many births. Her insides, now hanging out, were encrusted with flies. She looked at me, for just a moment, then walked to a corner to compete for a spot of shade. And for every animal that wasn't in extreme distress, there were dozens who were simply scared and in their last weeks or months or days of life.

I went to my rental truck to take a break and look at the footage so far, to make sure everything was okay. I had just climbed in when I heard a door slam. Two men in cowboy hats walked over to a pen full of goats, chatting in what sounded like Jamaican patois. They grabbed two goats by their back legs and walked them backward like they were pulling a wheelbarrow. The goats cried out as they stumbled, trying to keep up. The men then flipped them one at a time onto the truck and hog-tied them with duct tape. Tears rolled down my face as I listened to the sound of the goats crying—a sound which I learned is eerily similar to the crying of a human child. Over the course of that first day, I learned the sound of misery from many species. It was a cacophony of desolation and fear. And I realized, and the realization was like a swift kick in the gut, that I could have come any day, any moment, and this is what I would have found. Nothing was special or unusual about this day in this place. These things happened the day before and the day before that. And if I headed to the airport after finishing this sentence and stepped out of my rental car in San Angelo, it's what I would see today.

Several hours later as I was leaving, I walked back to one of the pens holding the Holstein babies. No one was around, so I put my hand out over the rail. Immediately, four calves were sucking on my fingers. I knelt down to look at them eye to eye and put my fingers through the chain-links to let them suckle. I dropped my head down to my chest and closed my eyes. I heard the auctioneer inside the ring rambling: "Umbabadbadadadabumbadatwotwentyfivetwo-twentyfivetwothirty"—I could hardly understand a word. I had heard auctioneers before at the state fair, and I pictured him sitting there, busting out of his shirt and suspenders with a giant belly and cowboy hat. That seemed to be the unofficial dress code. I decided to step in to the building to check out what was happening. My vision was spot on for the auctioneer. "Umbabadbadadada bum bada . . . eighteen-month-old Holstein heifers from Denton Farms . . . We'll start the bid at . . ." Young female dairy cows who have not yet had a calf, "heifers" as they are called, were being moved into the auction ring one by one with an electric prod and being sold off to the highest bidder. They were terrified.

People looked on in the audience dispassionately while a few men jotted notes and raised their bidder numbers. Groups of kids sat together in the stands, licking ice cream cones (the irony) and goofing off. I stopped for a moment and thought about how science-fiction-like the whole scene was: a species (us) buying, selling, using, abusing, then killing frightened, innocent other species, viewing and treating them as commodities. This could be a horror film somewhere on another intellectually and spiritually evolved planet—especially since there is so much scientific evidence that we do not need animal products in our diets at all, and in fact it's making us sick and destroying our planet. And all because we're too selfish and brainwashed to realize that giving up meat and dairy is a small sacrifice. All because we insist it's our God-given right. How did it come to be this way? Indifference was law here, "humanity" illegal.

Or maybe our culture is just too desensitized to violence in general. I'd spent years now coming to terms with how clueless I'd been during my McDonald's days, when I'd been completely unable to make a connection between a living animal and chicken nuggets.

When I got back in the rental car that day, I drove slowly off the property, pulled the car over, and wept. And over the next several days, I drove 2,000 miles, heading from one auction to another, filming one disgusting, enraging, horrific scene after revolting, angering, dreadful scene. In the evenings, I'd wrangle a vegan meal in yet another dusty town, usually a bean burrito *"sin queso, por favor"* in a Mexican joint, and stumble back to my hotel room. There, I'd crack open a beer and get on the phone. I'd call Doug, Gene, my mother, my sister, and my closest friends to cry and rant. "You can't even imagine," I'd often say, and then try to put some of the horror into words. To Gene I could say, "I know you know what it's like—how do I stay sane?"

As terrible as these situations were, the even greater horror was the understanding that this was going on all over the country, all the time. And I wasn't even witnessing a factory farm or a slaughterhouse. I wasn't following these tiny, confused calves to their veal crates, I wasn't watching the spent dairy cows shoved onto the kill floor. This misery—at an everyday livestock auction open to the public—was beyond comprehension.

When I stepped off the plane at Logan Airport in Boston and saw Doug, I broke down. It took weeks to recover from what I'd seen, and the images haunt me to this day. But I was there to bear witness, and so was the camera so others could as well. The images that have come from undercover work in stockyards, factory farms, and slaughterhouses have changed countless lives. I sent my footage to Gene, and he was able to use it during the congressional hearings on the Downed Animal Protection Act. Some of the video also made it into the film *Peaceable Kingdom*.

My dream had once included traveling the world with a documentary camera crew, but now it was showing that world what was wrong with our broken, morally bankrupt food system and what that means for our humanity, our planet, and the beings with whom we share this earth. And I know now that this is why I am here.

8

....

My Three Hundred
Chicken Roommates

Brandy was pulled from a dumpster as a tiny chick. His crime
was his gender.

Egg farmers large and small need hens, and they get them from
hatcheries. Thousands upon thousands of chicks are born each
day at these enormous operations. But the farmers and giant industries who buy the hatchlings from them are interested in only fifty
percent of those births: Male chicks are as unnecessary to the egg
industry as male calves are to the dairy industry. They are simply a
by-product and are treated as such. When the eggs hatch, workers
called "sexers" grab the chicks from a moving conveyor belt and
look to see whether the bird is male or female. It's done in seconds
because the belt moves so quickly, so sexing isn't always accurate.
The females are plopped back down onto the conveyer belt, their
beaks are seared off, they're punched by a needle for vaccination,
tossed into a shipping box bound for some industrial or "free-
range" egg-laying operation, and they then endure endless days of
laying, laying, laying until they're "spent," as the industry calls

them, and are killed. The males, though, are literally tossed out with the trash. And that's why if you look in the dumpsters behind egg factories, you'll see countless huge plastic bags filled with newly hatched chicks, suffocating to death on their first day of life. Or if it's an up-to-date operation, the males will be macerated—ground up alive—in a high-speed grinding machine, a sort of wood chipper for live chicks. They become fertilizer. This is what we support whenever we consume eggs—no two ways about it. Even the smallest "happy farms" order their egg-laying hens from these hatcheries, already sexed and soon ready to produce. I often say that there is more suffering in the egg industry than in any other form of animal farming. People on my tours always ask me which kinds of eggs are "okay to eat," organic, free-range, or cage-free? They usually don't like my answer.

Brandy was one of the lucky ones. He had been rescued from a dumpster before it was too late, and brought as a chick to a Pennsylvania farm animal sanctuary called Ooh-Mah-Nee. He grew up in its peaceful setting, where every morning the sanctuary directors, Jason and Cayce, called to him for his breakfast. Within seconds, Brandy would appear. He would allow them to stroke his shiny black feathers and even enjoyed a hug, resting calmly in a cradle of arms. His friendly, good nature allowed him the privilege of free roaming the farm, and whenever his name was called, Brandy would come a-runnin'.

After years of rescuing and providing refuge to hundreds of animals, Ooh-Mah-Nee closed its doors. Running a farm animal sanctuary is hard work, and so is keeping it funded. After months of phone calls and arrangements, Jason and Cayce moved their animals to other sanctuaries, and we welcomed many of them, including Brandy, now about nine years old. With tears in his eyes and Brandy in his arms, Jason introduced us to him and told us all about him. It was clear he loved him and was having a hard time saying good-bye. He was worried that Brandy might become depressed if we didn't give him the same attention and name recognition he had for all those years. We assured him that we would be thrilled to shower him with love and keep up the social interaction that Brandy so clearly enjoyed.

We immediately started up the morning greeting ritual by calling Brandy from the pig barn, where he slept at night with a small group of hens. Every morning he would come running out, stopping once he reached my feet to allow me to pick him up. He held perfectly still while I kissed his head, stroked his feathers, and gave him a squeeze before I put him down to enjoy his breakfast alongside the hens. Throughout the day, we'd stop and dote on him, often bringing him into the house for treats and one-on-one time. Doug and I just couldn't get over what an affable bird he was. We had other roosters, and some that we'd even call friendly, but Brandy would actually seek us out. On many mornings, he'd wake up at dawn, push his little body through the pig door, trot up to our house, and stare into our kitchen through the window in the back door. We'd let him in, always with a warm "Good morning, Brandy!" and he'd stand at my feet while I cut up some grapes into bite-size pieces for him—his favorite. Then Doug would start coffee while I prepared breakfast for the dogs (Mio, Frida, and Carli at the time) and a special bowl for Brandy who would eat right alongside them. It was such an incredible thing to witness. He loved canned vegetarian dog food, applesauce, and scrambled eggs from our hens, which we also fed to our dogs and many animals on special diets.

Then, while I whirred around the kitchen preparing to head out on the farm to start the day, Brandy would find his way over to one of the dog beds and enjoy a full-bellied nap. He was precious—and he was almost a decade old. The extra food and nap time were good for him, so Doug tiptoed as he cleaned up the kitchen.

After his midmorning nap, Brandy would head back outside to spend time with his hens and lead them around the farm. He was a real gentleman with the ladies and would stand guard as they pecked and wandered. Later in the day, I'd call him back to the house to see if he wanted to come in after I finished farm chores. I'd stand there with an enormous, giddy-with-love smile, watching his little black form leave his hens and make a beeline down the center path of the farm. He would sit next to me on the sofa while I worked at my laptop and returned phone calls from the day. I loved his company and the sweet sounds he made as I stroked his feathers.

Brandy even happily obliged requests to sit on a visitor's lap— sometimes he even jumped right up into one. He never minded being held, and many people wanted to hold him. For a lot of visitors who had never spent time with farm animals, a huggable, friendly rooster meant serious cognitive dissonance. But there it was: Roosters can be downright cuddly, and Brandy was the sweetest and brightest kind of living proof. I think he knew that he wore the badge for this honorable job, an ambassador for farmed animals, and he relished his role.

One special friend of Brandy's was Will, who was about eleven years old when he first started coming to WFAS. He met Brandy the first time he visited the farm with his parents. Since he was in a wheelchair, I placed Brandy in his lap to meet him, which just thrilled Will to death. For his part, Brandy gave every indication of being delighted to rest and cluck there for as long as Will wanted. After that, Will came back to the farm again and again with his family, just to spend time with Brandy.

■ ■ ■ ■

Several months after Brandy arrived, another remarkably friendly bird named Ophelia was brought to us. She's from the other end of the industrial chicken spectrum: she's a "broiler," bred solely for meat. She was discovered abandoned in a New York City fire truck—quite the mystery—and then taken to the CACC, which contacted us.

Back when Ophelia came, we were still often quarantining small new animals, like rabbits, chickens, and baby goats, in separate cages in our house. That first day I gathered Ophelia onto my lap to examine her, she tucked her legs under her, closed her eyes, and fell asleep, cooing and purring as young chickens do when they're cozy and tired. I left her there and sat for a while to let her sleep then gathered a blanket next to me on the floor and moved her over to it. She immediately woke up, stretched her white wings, and walked back over to the comfortable spot on my lap. I was so touched that I let her sleep until my legs went numb. I had already seen her walking around perfectly healthy, so I ruled out illness. I think she was simply craving the closeness and warmth of another being.

Ophelia stayed in our house for two more weeks as we awaited test results to confirm she wasn't carrying disease. During that time, she was rarely in her cage unless I was out on the farm. She followed me around the house seemingly interested in my every move, and if I got a chance to sit down, she'd jump right up on my lap to perch or snooze. I'd often look down at her and catch her staring right back up at me, head tilted with one eye fixed on mine. I wondered if she was trying to tell me something or if she was as pleased by my companionability as I was with hers. Regardless, we connected. There was just something about her and the way she acted specifically with me. Even now when I go out to see her, I feel like I'm visiting an old friend. She looks me in the eye and knows me, and when I say her name and encourage her to come to me, she does. I scratch her belly where she can't reach, due to her unnatural size, which prompts her to preen her reachable feathers and my hand as sort of a tickle response. She looks at me as I talk to her. And when I pick her up for a cuddle, I think she gets as much enjoyment from it as I do.

Ophelia is still with us, which is amazing considering "broilers" are bred to live only forty-five days, at which time they reach market weight. She's now five years old and living happily with a flock of "white birds" (our name for "broilers") and a friendly, crooked-beaked rooster named Cassidy.

But after two years on our farm and at eleven years of age, Brandy's heart gave out. He'd had a fight with a newly arrived rooster who had literally flown the coop. It was a horrible, unforeseen accident, but the fight had begun before any of us spotted it. Brandy was beaten up pretty bad. I knew from past experience that roosters can go into shock or sustain internal injuries from these fights, so I immediately treated him and left him to rest in our quiet guest bedroom. As the hours went on, he began to exhibit signs that he was not going to make it. I freaked out and did everything I could think of to save him. I injected a steroid called Dexamethasone that can reverse shock. I pumped his chest where his heart would be, and even gave him mouth-to-beak resuscitation when his little head slumped and he took his last breath. I screamed when I realized my efforts were hopeless, and doubled over sobbing. I held him in my arms and cried like a baby—I was inconsolable for days. And even though that was more than four years ago, I still miss him terribly, and sometimes I have flashbacks of a handsome black rooster trotting toward the house like he owns the place.

It was Brandy's loss that made me realize I had to learn how to deal with my grief better and not let it overcome me. I have to do that for my staff, so they can be consoled and move on, but equally important, I have to do it for myself so I can keep going. My crazy-passionate, cause-driven life came about because of my deep love and respect for animals, so of course I'm wrecked by their deaths, but I have too much to do for the other animals in our care and the ones out there who will never find sanctuary. In the end, though, you never really get used to losing friends.

When I got back to Boston after filming in Texas, I had a hard time focusing on work. I felt off-kilter, and my perspective had changed; my work was less important to me than it had been. Shortly after that trip, I began the most important job of my career—producing and directing a documentary for the Discovery Channel. But the enthusiasm I had felt when I landed the gig faded soon after I started. There were tight budgets and deadlines and stress between me and my coproducer and good friend Olympia.

During the writing, filming abroad, and the many weeks spent in the editing room, I would stop and reflect on how long it had taken me to get to this point. But now that I was there, I wondered if it was where I wanted to be. Stockyard scenes played in my head, as did my experience at Farm Sanctuary and the people I already felt so close to there. The work they were doing seemed far superior in terms of giving back to the world. I began to rethink my career. This was where I'd worked so hard to be: producing and directing documentaries and traveling to foreign lands—but neither my head nor my heart was ever fully engaged. My priorities had changed.

I became more miserable and couldn't wait for the show to be delivered and done. Right near the end of the process, Discovery Channel execs came in and added their touch, which consisted of laying a wall-to-wall bed of techno music and cheesy voice-overs. What little charm the project had was homogenized out. When it was finally over, I packed up my desk and declined other freelancing offers. I needed time to think, but the answer was ringing clear: I wanted to get a job at Farm Sanctuary and learn how to start a sanctuary of my own. "There is so much work to be done," I thought, "that there is room in every community to help more animals in need and advocate on their behalf."

Doug and I began to talk daily about it. "I'm committed to this cause," I told him. "And I hate to say it, but it looks like we're going to have to keep the long-distance thing going for a while longer." If I was going to try my hand at sanctuary life, I needed to leave my life in Boston and to live, work, and train at Farm Sanctuary, if they would have me. This time, the long-distance relationship wouldn't involve hopping between urban centers; it would mean five-hour bus trips for him from NYC to the sticks.

My Three Hundred Chicken Roommates

Doug, always sensible and stoic, took this in stride. He took me seriously but also asked the tough questions. "Are you sure you want to leave your career entirely? Maybe you could just take a hiatus and volunteer for a while?" And, "What if you get rid of the Boston loft only to discover that caring for farm animals isn't right for you? Are you sure you want to give up your great place and all your crazy neighbor friends?" He knew this meant challenging changes for his life, too, but he never tried to dissuade me. When he heard my answers, he knew this was what I Had to Do, and he understood why. There was no discussion of breaking up—that wasn't an option. Doug supported and respected my decision, and aside from the extra schlepping, it was no strain for him to do so.

That doesn't mean he wasn't scared. We both were. I'd spent years working terribly hard to get where I was in the production world, with a title and resume that could continue to offer better opportunities and a steady income. Was I really going to give that up to make just over minimum wage as an animal caretaker, doing manual labor in all kinds of weather? My freedoms as a free-lancer would be gone, and fun, spontaneous moments, like romantic weekend getaways, would be on hold, if not over for good.

I called Gene. "I'd like to make you an offer," I said, and told him that in exchange for housing and training at Farm Sanctuary, I'd work my butt off on the farm. "And I will do any kind of video work you need pro bono, and to sweeten the deal, Doug is willing to lend his editing skills. It's a package deal that we'll donate."

"This sounds great, Jenny!" he told me. "I'm going to have to talk it over with Susie, but I'll see what we can work out." This was a good deal for the farm, but it was easy to see why he had to discuss it. Unlike many positions that people can jump into with minimal training, farm sanctuary work is very specialized. Few people—especially back then—had experience in it, and training had to happen intensively on the job. The staff might not want to do all the work involved in training, just to see someone leave a year later. In this case, though, we would save the organization thousands by doing in-house videos, and I had a good excuse for being temporary: I wanted to use my knowledge to help more animals and educate more people. It was also clear that I was dead serious and committed to the cause. Fortunately, the powers that be agreed to the deal. As soon as Gene called me back, Doug and I started making arrangements. I bought plenty of secondhand Carhartts, jeans, and sweatshirts and a good pair of vegan boots. Then I left life as I knew it. Doug, meanwhile, bought a pair of boots himself and began arranging his editing schedule to accommodate three-day weekends. And he started doing push-ups.

Doug drove with me up to Watkins Glen to help me move in at the sanctuary and unload the rest of my stuff into a storage unit. When we arrived at Farm Sanctuary, we parked by the now-familiar People Barn, and Gene came out to meet us. He hopped in the car and directed us to what would be my home for the next year: an apartment in a cabin whose other room held three hundred or so rescued commercial layer hens. I set down my bags and took a deep breath, inhaling the aromas of wood, mice, straw, and chicken poop. Then I smiled. "It's perfect," I told Gene.

I initially worked as a feeder, bringing breakfast and dinner to the animals in the infirmary and all over the farm. Between meals I refilled waterers, hay, and feed cans; scrubbed dishes, buckets, and giant feed bowls; and cleaned the shelter kitchen, bathrooms, and infirmary pens. It was quite a different life from working hours on end on film shoots or in front of monitors and computer screens. It was so peaceful to walk along the dirt roads from coops to barns in the solitude of the country, no car alarms or police sirens or busy streets. Birds clucking and chirping, cows mooing, pigs snorting, fresh air . . . I was in paradise. It freed my busy head in ways I hadn't experienced in years.

My routine as a feeder was a laborious one, and the first couple of weeks it kicked my ass. I began each morning by preparing special meals for the animals in the infirmary and in the small sheds surrounding the shelter office building that would often house new animals that had arrived, goats, turkeys, ducks, small pigs—it changed all the time. My next stop was the turkeys; I'd hoist large troughs, open the grain bin, and compete with thirty or so anxious, chirping turkeys as I scooped their feed from bin to trough. Then I'd cross the road over to the grain silos to fill buckets with pelleted pig feed and carry them to the pig troughs. This was a challenging task for my upper body since the fence was high and it had to be done with accuracy or the feed would spill everywhere. As soon as grain hit metal, the pigs would come out of the barn to greet me. Some were already there in anticipation, using their snouts to knock my bucket off-balance—a fun game in the porcine set. I heaved bucket after bucket into the troughs, scratching a few heads in between. The pigs had a damp, pleasant smell, and I loved petting their bristly backs and kissing any available snouts while they snarfed up their breakfast. Next were the ducks, rabbits, and the many chicken coops around the farm—more walking, bucket carrying, pouring, petting, and kissing anyone (animal-wise) close by. Then I fed out hay. First stop: cows. Not used to close proximity with 1,000-to-2,000-pound animals, I performed this task carefully.

The Lucky Ones

Until I knew who was friendly and who wasn't, I'd slip in through the side door and head straight up the ladder into the hayloft, then throw down fifty-pound bales of alfalfa and timothy grasses, dust filling my ears and nose. With a quick swipe of my pocket knife, I'd cut loose the baling twine and break the bales into large flakes to stuff into racks inside and outside the barn, keeping my distance from the herd until I got to know them.

The sheep were next, and if they were in the barn when I needed to throw down hay, they were too impatient to wait for me to cut the bales open, so I'd have to wade through them to get to the bales. Even the shy ones participated in the gridlock of bodies, all competing to reach the hay. As I began breaking the bales apart and stuffing hay into racks, I could often feel myself being literally airlifted by a flock of fluffy animals, like a human pinball being shot around by marshmallow flippers. Then I headed over to the goats right next door. After throwing down their bales, I'd have to climb down and elbow into the fray, groups of goats climbing on top of the bales King-of-the-Mountain style while butting others in competition. They were crazy! So playful! Each with a distinct personality that they weren't afraid to show. I loved them all, well, except for TJ—presumably named after William Shatner's action-packed TV hero T. J. Hooker—who always went after me. One time TJ rammed me with his giant horns while I was filling the hay racks. He bruised the whole left side of my rib cage. Goats can be surly, though it's typically the ones who have had a horrible past. Still . . . that TJ. He could be quite a turd.

The hauling and lifting could be grueling, and my allergies were often at their worst (ugh, hay fever), but I knew if I could manage and tolerate the extreme elements that this would be the life for me. It was a good thing I'd gone to that South Boston gym so regularly; this job was a real workout. I stopped moving only when I went back to my cabin and sat down for lunch with my cats, Bella and Henry, whom I had adopted while in Boston. But before I had a chance to get too relaxed, I'd head back out on the farm to resume my chores.

One of my responsibilities was to remove, clean, refill, and replace each poultry waterer, which involved hauling five or ten gallons of water to and from each barn. This requires a steady gait if you want your pants to stay dry (which, believe me, you do in freezing cold weather). Sometimes this wasn't so easy for me, but I figured out ways to make it work and eventually built up my arm muscles to handle the load. One bitter cold day as I carried the sloshing buckets, frost crunching under my feet, a snot drip frozen to my lip, and a nose that felt and looked like a bright red Popsicle, I found a sense of peace with all the challenges of the work. I thought about the unimaginable discomforts of animals living in confinement in eye- and lung-burning, ammonia-laden factory farms and how miserable and desperate they were, day in and day out. That thought gave me all the motivation I needed. And I thought about how glad I was to be a part of a community of people who shared my feelings, working together for an organization that cared and advocated for farmed animals—and does a phenomenal job doing it. Then I completely wiped out on a patch of ice, which brought me down from this epiphany in a hurry. "Here's hoping tomorrow's warmer," I muttered to myself, and turned back to my task of refilling the fountain. My jeans and long underwear froze instantly against my skin.

Before I'd set foot at Farm Sanctuary, I was aware of a lot of farm animal issues, but living with animals who are victims of the industry made them tangible—literally. And Susie was always there with an answer to my questions. It was while I had my fingers deep in the neck of a sheep named Thelma, for example, that I wondered if there was a humane way to produce wool. I still had wool sweaters in my closet, many of which were my favorites. I may have been from the land of cheap synthetic fibers, but I liked a cozy wool sweater as much as anybody. And don't sheep *need* to be sheared? Why would you waste a product that comes from the clippings of the hair of an animal? No harm is done to them, right? What's the problem?

Alas, plenty.

"Once upon a time," started Susie, "people spun wool from the gently plucked tufts of molting sheep, animals whose natural fleece growth insulated them in summer and winter alike. No problem there." But somewhere along the way, farmers started genetically manipulating them through selective breeding.

Sheep grow enough wool to cover, insulate, and protect themselves. It is only through human involvement that the wool keeps growing, because it is constantly being sheared off. People have selectively bred our modern sheep to have thick, heavy coats. Sheep are sheared each spring, after lambing, just before they would naturally shed their winter coats.

Merino sheep, Susie told me, are by far the most common breed in Australia—the wool capital of the world—and they have it worst. They are bred to have wrinkled skin, like the shar-pei dog breed, meaning extra surface area of wool per sheep. But near their backsides, those wrinkles serve as breeding grounds for flies and maggots and contribute to a buildup of urine and feces. "So what do the farmers do? They slice big swaths of skin off, using knives or shears, in order to create patches of smooth scar tissue. The process is called 'mulesing.' And they do this, as you can probably guess, without anesthesia or painkillers of any kind," she said with disgust.

I felt sick. "So you're saying they're basically skinned alive?" I asked, my stomach tightening. I pictured someone restraining the family dog in a device that allows for little movement and, using gardening shears, cutting a large patch of skin from the dog's body. It's mutilation, and no less painful for the sheep—yet it's a common practice. Could anybody stand this? And would anyone even consider buying a product that supported that kind of direct cruelty to an animal? But people do, all the time—whenever they buy Merino wool as I had done myself.

If the animals survive this trauma, they are exposed yearly to the distress of shearing. "Because shearers are paid by the animal, not the hour, there's incentive to go as quickly as humanly possible," Susie explained. "I've seen everything, all sorts of gashes, and injuries from when they are flipped roughly over onto their rumps." When I looked into it further, it only got bleaker. According to one eyewitness, "The shearing shed must be one of the worst places in the world for cruelty to animals. . . . I have seen shearers punch sheep with their shears or their fists until the sheep's nose bled. I have seen sheep with half their faces shorn off. . . ." I was horrified.

Eventually most sheep from Down Under are shipped off on giant, multilevel ships bound for the Middle East and North Africa, where the ones who survive the arduous journey (usually without food or water) will be sold and slaughtered upon arrival. Some are bought at the dock where they are then bound up and thrown into the trunks of cars or in the backs of pickups. They are often kicked, beaten, and dragged off the boats by their ears and legs. They are then slaughtered at private homes, butcher shops, or unregulated slaughterhouses, where their throats are slit in front of one another while they are still conscious. It's a massacre, in countries where animal welfare standards are nonexistent.

Looking at their severely docked tails, the relationships between mothers and lambs, the friendliness and affection I witnessed in many sheep, I finally *really* understood why vegans don't wear wool.

But I also knew that the sheep at Farm Sanctuary had to be sheared, which led to my final question: "So what do you do here with the wool after you shear it off?" Susie gave me an impressive answer: The staff spread the tufts in the nearby woods for birds and other animals to pick up as nest material. Cool: recycling at its best.

It's amazing what we don't know about the origins of products as common as wool. But we have the responsibility as consumers to seek what industries try to hide. It starts with making simple connections, for instance, that wool comes from sheep and that a great deal of wool is manufactured. Huh . . . that must mean a lot of sheep. So how do they live? What is their daily existence like? What happens to them when they get old—or do they even get to grow old? It's a logical thought process, but one that we typically fail to follow to a conclusion, perhaps because of the commonality of wool, meat, and other things that come from animals. For those of us who claim to love animals, we have an obligation to examine what they must endure in order for us to enjoy such products—especially since these products aren't necessary for our warmth or health. Taking the time to look into and reconsider items made from animals allows us to make ethical decisions at restaurants and markets, at clothes stores and drug stores. Most people have no idea what they are supporting, so I don't look at them as heartless or barbaric; I know they are uninformed, and misled by false advertising, just like I had been for years. I fantasized about required truth-in-advertising labels like they have on Canadian cigarette packs—although instead of X-rays of cancerous lungs, they would show Merino sheep with their bloody backsides and include text like: *WARNING: This animal was mutilated and then shipped off for slaughter for this cardigan.*

It became clear to me that I needed to learn about caring for farm animals, but also to learn all there was to know about their lives and deaths so that I could advocate more effectively at my own sanctuary. And no matter what information came my way or what awful footage I was screening to produce a video, the blow was softened by the fact that I was living vegan and working on behalf of farm animals. We can do without animal products, so shouldn't the moral scale weigh on the side of compassion and nonviolence? The late Gretchen Wyler, actress and champion of animal rights and protection, once declared: "We must not refuse to see with our eyes what they must endure with their bodies." Right on, sister.

Some of the saddest realities of modern-day farming involve chickens. We have manipulated genetics to satisfy our greed, at the great expense of those animals. Now, caring for them daily and getting to know them, I saw this more clearly than ever. Before learning about the different sectors of the poultry industry, I'd always imagined that the same chickens were used for both eggs and meat. Not so, thanks to modern science. We have exploited genetics to get the most bang for our buck. The commercial poultry industry relies on only a few poultry breeds to produce hybrid broilers and layers, and those are the new standard "breeds" we've created in this country.

People like big juicy chicken breasts, so scientists engineered a Frankenbird of sorts, a "broiler" whose breasts are grotesquely enlarged. They are so immature when killed, the females haven't even begun to lay eggs. They are bred and drugged to grow so large, so quickly, that their poor legs and organs can't keep up; as a result, heart attacks, organ failure, and crippling leg deformities are common. Susie and I talked about their myriad health problems while I held a broiler hen so that Susie could treat and wrap her arthritic hock. I asked why they kept the hens separated from the roosters, and her answer surprised me.

"Well, with some birds like these guys and commercial turkeys that are bred to be unnaturally heavy, when males try to climb up on females, they are so enormous that they can break their backs. And they can rip the hens' fragile skin trying to use their claws and talons to scramble up. That's why chickens and turkeys have to be artificially inseminated: because of what we humans have done to them."

I shook my head and cursed quietly. Then I reached out and waited for a curious hen to waddle over and check out my outstretched hand.

My Three Hundred Chicken Roommates

Unbelievably, "broilers" grow so quickly that they are slaughtered when they're still babies, just over a month old. I'm actually glad that these birds have such short lives, considering the misery they endure. On the bright side (if you can call it that): Unlike commercial "layers," broilers' beaks aren't cut off, and the males aren't thrown into suffocating trash bags or ground up alive in a macerator. They are kept together because, at that age, they haven't reached sexual maturity, so there's no issue with related injuries. On the everything-else side: These birds are kept on the floors of enormous, dark sheds, thousands crammed into each, the ammonia of their waste burning their eyes and lungs, their overgrown muscle tissue—meat—causing them to become lame, hobble in pain, and often die when their legs give out and they can't make it to water or food.

Their birth to death is forty-five days. That's how far we've gone, how severely we've manipulated their genes. They reach around five pounds at six weeks of age, and that ain't normal. But compare that life with that of a "layer." Modern hens are bred to lay up to three hundred eggs a year, and we all know what's in those eggs—lots of protein, fat, and, in the shell, calcium for rigidity. Those nutrients don't come from thin air; they come from the poor hen who is pushing an object larger than her head through her nether region almost every day. (Some hens become "egg-bound" and die from being too weak to push another egg out of their bodies.) So if the hen isn't taking in enough calcium, for example, her body will leach it from her bones, and that's why so many layers are horribly disfigured in their cages, suffering from osteoporosis, broken bones, and paralysis. These birds live their whole life with at least four or five others in small wire enclosures known as battery cages, stacked row after row, as far as the eye can see, in massive industrial sheds: the quintessential factory farm. In the United States, ninety-five percent of hens used for laying live like that, and as of the end of 2008, there were 300 million hens living in battery cages—that's just about one for every U.S. citizen. Totally out of sight, therefore out of mind.

Like any animal, chickens are highly motivated to perform natural behaviors: in their case, nesting, perching, scratching, foraging, dust bathing, exploring, and stretching. But for up to eighteen months, day in and day out, they suffer unimaginable frustration because they are denied all of these behaviors, living shoulder to shoulder in a cage smaller than a file drawer. Doug gives his tours a visual that sums it up. He recalls being a child stuck in elevator at Macy's, him, his mom, a dozen perfume-wearing ladies, and a growing sense of claustrophobia. Those ten minutes had so much impact that he still remembers the feelings to this day, and yet that was just *ten minutes.*

When their time is up, the hens are yanked out of their cages by their legs and shoved into crates loaded on a trailer bed for their final destination. These "spent" hens are so scrawny and bruised they don't have the kind of meat that consumers would find palatable in a styrofoam tray, and so it's usually heavily processed for chicken soup, pet food, and other low-grade products.

A layer's life, then, is several times as long as that of her broiler counterparts, and even worse in terms of misery. No wonder vegans often feel that vegetarianism is more like a step along the way to ethical eating than a place to stay put, hard as that might be to comprehend at first.

So, since they're engineered to meet such specific needs, those birds can't stand in for each other. A laying hen is too slight to grow the large, muscled breasts that consumers demand. That's why the males born at layer hatcheries don't get sent off to Perdue but rather are killed outright. And a broiler will never be able to produce the eggs that a company like Safeway demands.

Sharing a house with hundreds of spent layers one door away made me hyperaware of the lives they lived before their rescue. All were debeaked, some so severely that it was painful to look at them. But they were the lucky ones, who had been rescued from a tornado-devastated factory farm in Ohio. Tens of thousands of others at that facility perished, either in the storm or when they were bulldozed along with the other wreckage during the "cleanup." Now they were living beautiful, happy lives at Farm Sanctuary, but those lives were much too short. Some suffered from cysts, infections, and others from ovarian carcinoma and other diseases of the reproductive tract. They were valued only for their production levels, and were pushed beyond their biological limits; the odds were against them from the very beginning.

Before long, I'd proven myself at Farm Sanctuary, so health care duties were added to my daily roster of chores. Now I was learning how to vaccinate, trim pig hooves, salve joints, wrap feet, splint limbs, disperse meds, administer IV fluids, and more. I was even helping Susie tether pigs and cut their tusks, which made me flash back to the first day I'd set foot at the sanctuary, when I'd heard chilling pig screams and watched Susie handle poop with her bare hands.

The pigs, primarily because of their gargantuan size, were

endlessly challenging and sort of hilarious to deal with. Christopher-Pig, for example, needed his foot dressing changed every single day. He had a chronic infection he just couldn't shake. Christopher weighed somewhere around a thousand pounds, and at least a hundred of those had to have been in the leg we had to deftly handle. The procedure took two people—one to give him a distracting belly rub and one to change the dressing. Sounds simple, right? My arm muscles felt like they were going to peel off the bone from those belly rubs! And if I was playing the wound-dresser role, that meant somehow hefting that hock up, often onto my fake foot, which could handle the weight a lot better than my real one, and steadying it for bandaging. It was quite the operation.

Another "fun" medical job was dealing with the many hens who had a condition called egg peritonitis. It's really sad, actually. Egg-laying hens are engineered to lay such an artificially large number of eggs that one can sometimes get stuck in the tract. Unfortunately, by the time the problem's noticeable, there's just no way to fix it. First, chickens don't do well under anesthesia, and that's what would be needed to attend to this serious a problem. Second, part of the egg has usually attached itself to the oviduct, or the hen has prolapsed and pushed out her reproductive tract. But we spent enough time with the chickens to recognize the signs: A hen with egg peritonitis starts to walk funny because the blockage causes a lot of fluid to build up behind the egg. Our job, then, was to drain that fluid every day to relieve the discomfort. I'd first mark the hen with a dab of color on her back to make it easier to find her in the flock during the coming days. Then I'd gather her into my arms, position her butt over a measuring container in the sink, swab a spot on her abdomen with alcohol, and use a large-gauge needle (without a syringe attached) to slowly drain up to two cups of stinky fluid from her belly. It wasn't unusual for a hen to relax and fall asleep in my arms; she'd be so relieved from the release of pressure. When Doug was visiting I'd give him the job of holding the hen, and when the smell wafted up he would struggle to contain the contents of his stomach!

As one can imagine, my lifelong, deep-seated fascination with gross things really served me well at Farm Sanctuary. To me, lancing abscesses was enjoyable. To this day, squeezing turkey pimples (they're infected feather follicles, actually) is an obsession. And treating bumblefoot, which means peeling the scab off an infected chicken foot, removing the hardened pus plug, squeezing out the fresh pus, and irrigating the wound? Very satisfying. It's disgusting, I know. Even Susie was impressed at how much I genuinely liked the gross-out jobs. She was and is exactly the same way—yet another reason I love her. It got to the point where she'd call me on my walkie-talkie and tell me to head over if she was embarking on a disgusting procedure.

Health care for farm animals is not as straightforward as it might sound. This kind of "care" is traditionally about keeping an animal's heart beating just long enough for "it" to walk to untimely slaughter. We were asking vets to help us deal with ailments that they had sometimes never even seen, let alone treated. When a chicken isn't expected to live more than forty-five days and you're asking a vet to treat her arthritis, you know you're in uncharted territory. Ditto for uterine cancer in an elderly goat or a 2,000-pound steer with spinal tumors.

Even common ailments that occur within animals' average factory-farm life span aren't usually identified or treated. If a farmer does notice, depending on the species, there's little incentive to spend the time, money, and energy treating animals for curable ailments. For example, there's no way most people involved in factory farming could diagnose egg peritonitis until a hen has died of the condition. But we who do this work—and the supporters who provide our funding—see large and small ailments as issues worthy of the same treatment we'd give dogs and cats—or humans, for that matter, and we do everything we can to treat ailments, relieve pain, and hope for survival.

If a vet had an "It's just a chicken" attitude, we'd protest and take our money elsewhere. But to their credit, many of the vets we contacted were game to try procedures they'd never been taught in vet school. There was sometimes some initial head scratching or questioning, but they were able to make the perspective shift without much trouble. The most enthusiastic were at Cornell, which was, fortunately enough, only an hour away from Farm Sanctuary. Cornell has long been renowned for its veterinary program, and the staff members there are often up for new teaching opportunities. The avian vets might be used to treating canaries and cockatoos, but they don't often see someone bring a ten-dollar turkey into their practice for a $400 surgery. Even for willing experts it was a medical challenge, no question. They worked by drawing on their knowledge of similar procedures and cases and doing their best, which generally worked just fine. Unfortunately, Cornell never offers free or discounted service to our charitable organization, which has always irked me—especially since it is a teaching hospital and the students learn so much from our cases.

My Three Hundred Chicken Roommates

....

Doug, now back in Manhattan, came faithfully via a five-hour bus ride almost every weekend. It meant a demanding dual life for him, but he loved being in the country and helping me care for the animals. And besides, we missed each other a lot. He was finding it fun to get out of the city and realize a radically different way of life. It opened his mind—and his heart. He would come in on a Friday evening, and I would pick him up at the bus station in Ithaca, forty minutes away. If I wasn't on call at the farm that evening, we'd often have a romantic dinner in town and crash from full bellies and long days when we got back to the farm. We were used to spending our weeks apart by then, but now I would often have to work one or both weekend days, so our time was even more limited. While I was working, he would edit a Farm Sanctuary video or one of the projects that he brought up from the city, like episodes of Comedy Central's *Insomniac with Dave Attel*, while hens cooed on the other side of the wall. But Doug didn't just stay chained to his monitor; he did his share outside, too. He'd sometimes wake up early and start feeding the pigs while I was still filling troughs at one of the chicken houses. He had his limits, though. He categorically stayed away from the gross stuff. He didn't even want to be in the same barn while I lanced abscesses, and he would rarely hang out in the med building, where he might walk in on something he wasn't prepared to see. But he enjoyed the chores and loved not only hanging out with the animals but also the new definition in his biceps. It all made for a satisfying counterpoint to hour upon hour of editing digitized video.

In the evenings, if we had any energy left, we'd make dinner together in the little cabin kitchen. We were becoming experts at preparing satisfying, yummy, stick-to-your ribs vegan food—burritos, pizza, pasta, shepherd's pie, tamale pie, casseroles. We wanted for nothing. These days we're apt to make more complex gourmet dishes (when we have time!), but those days were slightly before the burst of vegan products and resources that have flooded the market since. And back then, we were just learning all that a vegan diet had to offer. Still, we ate well, and it was fun to explore our new gastronomic world. We took a lot of trips to the little health food store in Watkins Glen to make discoveries and experiment with ingredients. In addition to the delicious premade egg-less egg-salad sandwiches we always grabbed to eat on the car ride back, that store introduced us to new convenience foods—like Tofurky deli slices and even soy beef jerky—and new (to us) grains, quinoa and amaranth among them. And when we visited Ithaca, we'd go nuts shopping at the mecca of natural, organic, community-owned food co-ops, GreenStar. We perused vegetarian cookbooks and successfully experimented with veganizing the recipes with no trouble at all. And we swapped recipes and cooking tips at frequent potlucks at Gene and Lorri's and the homes of other staff.

....

9

Woodstock, a Wedding, and a Band of Turkeys

Turkey Poults for Sale," read the ad in a local paper in Binghamton, New York. An entrepreneurial yet inexperienced hobby farmer had placed the classified, looking to unload young turkeys for cheap. He was failing miserably at raising them to sell for Thanksgiving. Many had fallen ill and were dying left and right, but instead of seeking veterinary help, he weeded out the healthy ones to sell and salvage something from his investment while he still could. Boone, Alphonso, and Herschel, along with the remaining eighty-plus baby turkeys, were being sold for seven bucks a pop.

A woman from a local animal rescue group called the farmer, incognito, claiming to want to buy some. When she arrived at the man's house, she took one look at the birds' poor condition and the dirty, unheated garage they were living in and offered to take them all off his hands. Surprisingly, he accepted, saying, "I think I got a bad batch." He admitted that he was in over his head. He had no Internet to search for guidance and didn't want to invest any more time, energy, or money into the turkeys' care.

The Lucky Ones

Within two weeks, all had been quarantined and treated for parasites at Farm Sanctuary and then welcomed at homes and sanctuaries alike. We took in three boys, or "toms," and they grew up here, an inseparable trio. (Two are still here now, six years later—that's simply ancient for commercially bred turkeys.)

Besides escaping with their lives, Boone, Alphonso, and Herschel were lucky in another way: Unlike ninety-nine percent of turkeys raised in the United States, they hadn't been debeaked, detoed, and desnooded without anesthesia or pain remedies—savage procedures done to cut down on fighting injuries. For the non–turkey experts out there, the snood is that red droop of flesh over a turkey's beak. (Doug tells his tours they were invented by Dr. Seuss, and I think about half of them believe him.) Workers tear them off turkeys' faces with their fingers. Then they snip off the end of their toes with clippers and place their sensitive beaks in the same kind of slicing machine egg-laying hens are subjected to, leaving many to die from the trauma. As is standard, there is absolutely no regard for their pain, but their feed is laced with antibiotics to combat infections from the wounds.

Like all domesticated turkeys raised for meat, Boone, Alphonso, and Herschel were genetically compromised from the start, bred to grow massive in a short time so that they could be killed when they were only fourteen to eighteen weeks old. Because of their inability to reproduce naturally due to their enormous breasts, a male turkey has to be "milked"—i.e., masturbated—at a production facility and his semen collected into vials. Then, in another facility, the females used for breeding are turned upside down, their legs are spread apart by shackles, and they are artificially inseminated with an instrument similar to a turkey baster. It's essentially turkey rape with a foreign object, and it's just wrong on all kinds of levels.

If similar mutilations and practices were imposed on cats and dogs, there would be public outrage. But the majority of people don't realize it's happening to the animals that land on their plates, or stop to think what animals go through before they're eaten. A turkey, like any other creature with a nervous system, experiences pain, which is, after all, a survival mechanism. But if people did know, would there be the same outrage?

■ ■ ■ ■

Our three boys accepted us into their flock, waddling all around the farm, following us wherever we went. They liked the company and were curious about everything we were doing. Back then we were still fencing, digging out three-foot-deep holes every ten feet, stopping to pry rock after rock out of each hole. The turkeys loved this activity—so much so that they made our work difficult by constantly getting in the way to see what bugs we might have unearthed. But all the activity helped keep their weight down. I knew from my time at Farm Sanctuary that I had to compensate for their massive weight and fragile frames by making sure they got plenty of exercise, along with a very low-fat, fiber-rich diet full of fruits and veggies. Boone, Alphonso, and Herschel said thank you for their healthy lives by being three of the most extroverted, loving animals on the farm.

Boone is the most social, always underfoot, following staff around or blocking the way into a barn or building. He'll chirp at the back door of the medical center, where his special food is kept, for hours. The other turkeys eat a particular grain mix as their staple, but Boone has an abnormality. His tongue stays down in his throat, resting visibly in his neck below the jaw instead of in his mouth. This, as you can imagine, makes it hard for him to eat: He takes a bite of food, then lifts his head to bite at air, his snood flopping around his head like a flaccid baton as he chirps and swallows. So to make it easier on Boone, he gets a delicious mash made of grains, applesauce, veggies, and fruit blended with water—his premier joy in life. No one has found a time when Boone doesn't think he needs another mash. While he's working on his bowlful, he usually steps in it with his giant feet. He gets mash on his head, in his nose, and all over his face. He has a voracious appetite. Take the laundry out, there's Boone. Bring one of the med building residents, say an ailing chicken, outside for the afternoon, there's Boone. Bring the chicken back in at dusk, Boone. Call out "Boone!" and he pulls his feathers close to his body for better aerodynamics and comes running. If he slips into the med center behind someone and there's no mash, he pushes his chest against their legs, stretches out his neck, and chirps his pleas as they try to mix up a batch. We have to monitor how much we give him, naturally, but his tongue anomaly is actually a saving grace in keeping his weight down. But it's hard to resist his pleas for more.

A couple of years ago, we had a big scare; Boone got a virus that almost killed him. He became listless and weak, lost weight, and was starting to lose the spark in his eyes. He slept for hours on piles of blankets in his pen in the med center, lying motionless in the boat shape that a turkey takes when he sleeps—head tucked under a wing and feet folded underneath. What worried us more than anything was that he wouldn't eat his mash. Since turkeys aren't treated the same as dogs and cats, we were on our own in trying to figure out how to help him. After days on his prescribed medications, syringe feeding, poking him with needles to administer fluids, and lots of hand-wringing and worry, Boone sat up, starting chirping, and excitedly pecked at the bowl of food presented to him. Boone was eating! He was back! There was an enormous collective sigh of relief around the farm. And after a week or so, besides losing a few pounds, Boone was back to his old self and probably now holds the record for number of times a turkey has been kissed on the head.

Alphonso is a more mellow turkey, less charismatic and outgoing than Boone, but friendly and sweet. Where Boone will grab a treat out of your hand, Alphonso will gently take it. Where Boone will stretch his neck out and move around while you try to hug him, Alphonso will relax his body into yours and engage in a hug and enjoys having his feathers and chest stroked gently. He loves to strut around, poufing and vibrating his feathers. It makes him look serious and handsome. He has especially overgrown, callused feet that we soak regularly as therapy and often have to wrap. Between his poor feet and his snood, he looks a mess.

Boone might be Alphonso's best friend, but they get on each other's nerves sometimes—especially during mating season when hormones flare. When they were younger, they would jump and try to claw and kick each other (hence the toe chopping at the hatcheries). Their fights were brutal, and we'd have to run out to separate them. Even now, they sometimes peck furiously at the other's face: Alphonso's scarred snood tells the tale. But they're always together despite their skirmishes, the Odd Couple of the farm.

Herschel was quiet, too. He was a different kind of turkey: a Bronze. He looked more like a wild turkey than the usual white bird of today's farms. (Turkeys—and commercial "broiler" and "layer" chickens—have the color genetically bred out of their feathers in the quest for whiter-looking meat and eggs. The darker pin feathers—those with a blood supply—are considered "unattractive" when the carcass is "dressed.") Herschel was one of those "heritage breeds" that breeding associations try to preserve for the sake of "conservation" and a niche "natural" item to market, unsightly pin feathers and all. He was covered in beautiful dark feathers that took on an iridescent green and copper sheen when the sun hit them. But he was even more genetically overgrown than his white-feathered counterparts. He tipped the scales at forty-plus pounds at one point, leading us to put him on an especially restrictive diet. It's trendy for consumers to buy conservation breeds, but as natural as people might want the turkeys to be for health or conscience, the producers want the same ten extra pounds when it comes time to sell them by weight. Consumers don't realize that these birds are still genetically manipulated for profit. There's nothing really natural about it.

Herschel enjoyed a massage on his bright, rubbery head, or just having someone sit down next to him. He liked to look up into my face and make eye contact while I stroked his feathers. Herschel, Boone, and Alphonso were dubbed the Three Wise Men. They traveled as a pack, poufing out their feathers, strutting and following us around for the morning feedings and during our tours on the weekends. They were hilarious. Visitors marveled at their bond, how they mimicked one another's movements, and the way they sometimes made figure eights while strutting and chirping.

Woodstock, a Wedding, and a Band of Turkeys

On his tours, Doug warns the visitors not to be fooled: This band of turkey comrades is operating a sophisticated racket where one distracts you while the other two nab your wallet and run your Visa card. It would be a great way to stay funded, but, alas, it is patently false.

A few friends have chosen to have their weddings here at the farm, and on more than one such special occasion, the three turkeys followed the bride and groom down the aisle, poufing away in their feathery finery. Since then, sweet Petunia, one of our female turkeys, followed another couple to the altar, much to their delight.

The Three Wise Men posse's effect on people was really profound. I remember one family who visited a couple of years ago, a husband and wife with two small children. The woman was already vegetarian and wanted to make some connections for her family, but her husband, though plenty curious and happy to be there, was mostly along for the ride. As we toured the farm together, Boone, Alphonso, and Herschel tagged along as usual. Boone walked right up and demanded attention, cocking his head in curiosity. The family was surprised and amused by his personality and lack of apprehension—especially the husband. He'd been hanging back a bit, quiet, but I could see him gaining an interest in Boone. He knelt down in front of him and reached out a hesitant hand. Boone inspected his palm, hoping for food, then gently pecked at his shiny gold watch. The man laughed and stood up but kept watching Boone as we walked and the turkeys kept following. I took them to meet the chickens, goats, sheep, and steer before stopping outside the pig barn to watch them eat. All the while, the Three Wise Men tagged along. The husband reached for Boone's head to stroke him and feel his feathers while Boone stood still, looking up at him.

The Lucky Ones

At the end of the tour, the man turned to his children and said, "Guys, I'm ashamed." He explained that he'd always assumed that turkeys were dumb and didn't possess individuality or personality. He had thought of them only as deli slices and the Thanksgiving meal centerpiece. But it was obvious after spending the afternoon with the birds, he said, that they weren't the dumb birds he had imagined. "They're smart and friendly—I never imagined," he told his kids, and declared that he could never eat (a) turkey again. Weeks later, his wife sent us an e-mail telling us that she couldn't believe the change that had come over him, and that he'd kept his word: He had stopped eating turkeys, and all animals, in fact, and so had the kids—theirs was now a completely vegetarian family. She was impressed that we had the gumption to go against the grain and ask people to reconsider their relationship with and attitude toward farm animals. And though the information about animals raised for food is painful to hear, she knew it was important to hear. Boone, Alphonso, and Herschel, like all the animals in our care at WFAS, are ambassadors for our cause. When people meet them and see how personable they are, it's harder to turn around and ignore the lives of their equals languishing around the world.

Turkeys may very well be the most misunderstood of all farm animals. Have you heard the saying, "How can I soar with eagles when I work with turkeys?" People actually disparage turkeys for being "too dumb" to fly. But they *can't* fly—though instinct urges them to. Wild turkeys can, but the ones bred for eating have bodies absurdly big for their own wings and can only dream of flying, frustrated and stressed from their efforts. Turkeys have been flying for millennia—it's sad but understandable that their domestic cousins want to do that, too. I'd hardly question their intelligence as a result.

Woodstock, a Wedding, and a Band of Turkeys

But animal behaviorists and poultry scientists don't doubt their IQ. "I've always viewed turkeys as smart animals with personality and character, and keen awareness of their surroundings," says Tom Savage, a poultry scientist at Oregon State University. "The 'dumb' tag simply doesn't fit." Researcher Jo Edgar, at the University of Bristol, said of chickens, which have intelligence similar to that of other poultry, like turkeys: "We found that adult female birds possess at least one of the essential underpinning attributes of empathy—the ability to be affected by, and share, the emotional state of another." Birds like chickens and turkeys can anticipate future events based on the past and use their judgment accordingly, and they have complex intercommunication.

People also don't associate poultry with mothering skills, but ground-nesting birds, like turkeys and chickens, have a very strong mother-chick bond. In fact, a turkey mom starts chirping to her chicks while they're still in the egg, to accustom the babies to her voice. Once hatched in nature, chicks sleep under their mother's wings every night and are gathered for warmth and comfort periodically during the day. If a poult gets lost, he or she will panic and begin peeping like mad. The mother will respond by running after the poult and gathering the chick under her wing.

We lost Herschel in 2009. He was not as successful as his friends at overcoming the problems of genetic modification. Despite plenty of exercise and carefully measured feedings of grain, vegetables, and fruit, he couldn't comfortably support his own weight, and he developed crippling arthritis in both of his legs. We tried physical therapy and a variety of salves and medications suggested by the vet, but nothing worked. When his pain became too much and he could no longer walk, we gave him a special meal, showered him with hugs and kisses, and drove him to the vet to be peacefully euthanized in my arms. The Three Wise Men became two, and it was obvious from Boone's and Alphonso's movements and moods that they missed their third. So do we. Now other rescued turkeys have joined Boone and Alphonso in their adventures around the farm: Petunia, Sphinx, Beatrice, and Timmy and Tommy—and there have been others whose lives were cut short like Herschel's, in spite of our best efforts.

With almost a year at Farm Sanctuary under my belt, Doug and I felt it was time to get going on our own ambitions. We were engaged by this time—he had proposed to me one evening in a beautiful hilltop cow pasture at Farm Sanctuary. We were ready to begin our lives together and were fully committed to starting a sanctuary of our own, and I felt, and still feel, that with Doug by my side, everything was possible. It was a scary prospect to start our own sanctuary, but every cell of my being wanted and needed to do it. I had my own vision and drive, and I wanted to bring a haven to another area to help more animals and educate others about their plight.

We said good-bye to all the people and animals that we had grown to love at Farm Sanctuary. I packed my things, leaving many of them in a storage unit not far from the sanctuary, and moved into Doug's apartment on the Upper West Side of Manhattan. Although he tried to convince me it was large by New York standards, it seemed tiny to me, though it had the advantage of being very close to Central Park. Our dog May, whom we had found running along the side of a highway during my time in Watkins Glen, and my cats, Bella and Henry, whom I had adopted in Boston a year or so after losing Boogie, would have to deal with life on the sixteenth floor. May was geriatric and Bella was a homebody, but poor Henry had grown accustomed to roaming all day and evening around the grounds at Farm Sanctuary. Now we supervised him as he wandered the long hallway lined with fourteen identical apartment doors, and he would go to the farthest one and roll around on the carpet and purr. He seemed to be saying, "Which one of these things leads back to the farm?"

During the week, Doug worked with Morgan Spurlock on the pilot episode of the series *30 Days,* while I stayed at home searching property listings and studying up on how to start a successful nonprofit. This venture was going to take time, money, know-how, and a solid plan, but it had to begin with an address. We wanted a parcel close to New York City, so that we could attract weekend visitors and Doug could continue his editing gigs to bring home the "soy bacon," as he likes to say. But the land had to be far enough away that we could acquire acreage and a house without paying an arm and my other leg.

With our budget and our criteria set, I hopped on Realtor.com. I started by looking for existing farms to buy—or at least a property with a house and a barn or two, enough acreage, and the right zoning. I'd scout appealing prospects, and then on the weekends, Doug would join me in visiting the most promising ones. We began by looking around western Massachusetts, where I knew the concentration of colleges would mean great visibility and a strong base of supporters and volunteers (and oh, how I love Northampton). But we couldn't afford squat there. We tried the eastern Hudson Valley next, over the Massachusetts border, but we couldn't find enough open acreage anywhere near civilization, which was critical to drawing in visitors and, on a personal level, keeping our sanity.

Then one winter day, after I'd looked at half a dozen properties, a lovely realtor named Blanca swung me into the driveway of 35 Van Wagner Road in Willow, New York, a hamlet outside the legendary town of Woodstock. We'd been watching this place from our computer for months. The original asking price had been way too high for us, but it kept dropping, and pending sales kept falling through. We wondered why, but it looked so gorgeous online and the location was so perfect—just a two-hour drive from New York City and in a town that already drew visitors—that when the price got (sort of) within range, I decided I had to check it out.

Blanca parked the car a little way from the house so that I could get a good look at the land. There were no barns or sheds, just acre after acre of raw, tan fields patched with snow, and toward the back a quirky gabled house that looked as though it had fallen from the sky onto the flat land, like the one in *The Wizard of Oz*. I climbed out of the car and checked out the surroundings. Thick woods fringed the fields, and behind the trees the Catskill Mountains rose soft and brown in panoramic views. It was a magical spot, and even knowing how much work would have to go into transforming it for our needs, I was in love. The farm seemed to build itself in my head. I could see a center path, barns on either side, coops and fences. Then we walked inside the house, and I stood in awe: Majestic two-hundred-year-old beams, cathedral ceilings, an open kitchen perfect for vegan feasts—I snapped picture after picture of every detail. It needed a roof and some updates from the use of mauve in the 1980s (it still does), but I pulled out my phone. It was useless, of course. No cell service here. But on my way back home I finally picked up a signal. "Doug!" I practically shouted. "I think this is the one!"

The owner had resisted selling—hence the repeatedly sabotaged sales—because the house was tied up with the end of his marriage. But by the time Doug and I came around for a second visit, he realized that he needed to go through with it and had begun packing. So, after an inspection, price negotiations, a heart-in-our-mouths deposit, and reams of thirty-year-mortgage paperwork, the place was ours. Thank god we got in before the bottom fell out of the mortgage business; these days I think a bank would look at our finances and then escort us out of the office. Neither of us had ever owned a home, and suddenly, we were in charge of sixteen acres of weedy fields, five acres of rusty-appliance-and-junk-car-filled woods, and a little under two acres for the *Wizard of Oz* house.

The high of first-time home-and-farm ownership couldn't last too long, though. There was so much to do. Doug was still working full-time, so a lot of the moving in and planning fell to me. We closed on the house in May, just six months after leaving Farm Sanctuary. After getting the house in order, we immediately got to work building our first chicken coop while a contractor worked on a new roof for the house. Hammers and drills rang and buzzed throughout the day. Meanwhile, we formed a board of directors and wrote our mission statement and bylaws in order to apply for nonprofit status. We also began a lengthy application process with the town that would allow us the right to eventually open our doors to the public. This was not easy. There were issues on how to classify us within the existing zoning laws: Were we a cultural facility?

The Lucky Ones

A farm? A nonprofit recreational facility? The process was absurd and dragged on for months. Although we were allowed to have farm animals in our particular zoning, we were in a residential district, which meant we had to apply for a special-use permit so that people could visit the farm. That meant endless meetings with the town's zoning board of appeals and planning board. It was a grueling, time-consuming, and complicated process, but we had to gain a status that would allow us to advertise public hours and welcome visitors.

At the same time, we began seeking volunteer help from friends, animal advocacy groups, and locals. Luckily, we had friends helping out from day one. We'd met a wonderful couple from the Woodstock area, Chris Kerr and Kirsti Gholson, way back at the Critter Care Conference at Farm Sanctuary and stayed in touch. Among Chris's many talents is building, and he was instrumental in the construction of our chicken coop, teaching Doug building techniques and how to handle tools along the way. Then there was our dear friend Sheila Hyslop, whom I had also met at Farm Sanctuary while she was doing an internship all the way from Scotland. When she learned that we had bought our land and were raring to go, she came back to the States and stayed with us for months to help. (Years later we coaxed her into applying for a work visa with us as her sponsor. She is now our legally permitted farm manager, with endless energy, commitment, and love for our animals, and the source of endless amusement about the funny way those Scots talk. Flashlights are now called "torches." Anything small is "wee.") Our friends Dan Piraro and Ashley-Lou Smith, die-hard animal activists whom we'd met at a Farm Sanctuary event, were also excited to come up from Brooklyn to help out. They became founding board members along with Kirsti and the wonderful Libra Max, the daughter of artist and animal rights champion Peter Max. Andy Glick, who ran the Woodstock Animal Rights Movement (WARM) store and organization in Woodstock, allowed us, with official documentation, to begin taking tax-deductible donations under his nonprofit umbrella. These wonderful people enabled us to literally hit the ground running.

Our new chicken coop filled with residents quickly. Rio, a rooster found on the streets of New York City, was our very first resident. His rescuer was keeping him in her city apartment but needed to find him a home before her neighbors complained. A series of calls led her to us, and Chris and Kirsti offered to foster him in their house in Woodstock (an experience they loved) while we readied the coop. Soon after Rio's entrance came a group of hens rescued from the Buckeye Egg Farm, an enormous factory farm with a national reputation for environmental irresponsibility and inhumane practices.

When tornadoes touched down and ravaged the town of Croton, Ohio, where Buckeye is based, several of the farm's warehouse buildings were destroyed. Inside those warehouses were more than a million egg-laying hens confined to wire battery cages that were stacked row upon row. For them, there was no warning that tornadoes were coming and no chance of escape. Twelve of the chicken warehouses were leveled. When the buildings' sides and roofs blew down, cages were mangled and many birds were instantly killed, but most were trapped helplessly, languishing without access to food, water, or medical attention. The owners decided the best way to deal with the damage was to just bulldoze the sheds filled with hundreds of thousands of trapped birds, the living among the dead. But after a lot of noise from rescue groups, the farms begrudgingly allowed rescuers to come *one day* and save those they could before the leveling.

Devastated by what they saw but undaunted, rescuers saved as many lives as possible. Five thousand hens were saved, and Farm Sanctuary became home to 1,200 of them—many of whom I lived next door to while I was there.

Since we didn't have not-for-profit status yet and were using our own limited funds to get started, we couldn't take in a huge number of birds, but we could start by taking in six. Here, they could continue to enjoy their new lives outside a cramped cage, with grass under their feet, perches and heat lamps at night, and all the sunshine and dust baths they could handle.

When the hens arrived, we opened their transport cages and watched them toddle tentatively onto the soft ground in front of their coop. I beamed as they flapped their wings, explored their new home, and interacted with one another. This was both a familiar and a new experience. I'd witnessed such introductions while at Farm Sanctuary, but now these little lives were entirely our responsibility. For all of them, each an individual with needs, this was home, a safe home where they would be loved.

Not long after finishing the chicken coop, we received more calls to take in chickens found in the New York City area, and it seemed new birds were arriving weekly. Then we got word about three steer who had been rescued as veal calves on a dairy farm. They had lived at another sanctuary for the first two years of their lives but were then adopted into a home that proved an irresponsible one. Libra Max, their original rescuer, wanted them out of there since their safety was at risk, and she was none too happy with the sanctuary that had placed them. She reached out to us to see if we were willing to take them in, offering to help financially to make it happen. Immediately we got to work fencing a few acres, then bought a run-in shed, a three-walled structure, to shelter them. So in our first year on the land we welcomed three handsome young steer, whom Libra had named Ralphie, Elvis, and Andy.

When they first came, the trio loved to find ways to get out of their pasture. One winter night when I was home alone, the steer climbed a snowdrift and stepped right over their fence. I was panic-stricken and terrified they would run into the road and get hit by a car. I began frantically searching around the farm. "How far could they have gone?" I wondered. "Are they destroying someone's yard? Heading into the woods?" I calmed down long enough to devise a plan. I tore open a fifty-pound bag of "sweet feed" (their favorite thing in life) and poured it into the back of the pickup, then drove around listening and looking for the boys. Once I spotted them, merrily grazing on the side of the road, I pulled up alongside, hoping they would pick up the scent of the feed. It worked. All three rushed to the truck bed and followed me as I picked up speed and drove back to the farm and through the fields to their pasture (thank God for four-wheel drive). I was proud that I had succeeded in getting the trio of steers back all by myself, but from then on I tried to make sure I was never on my own at night—and that we managed the snowdrifts until we could get an electric line set up that would prevent such escapes. It was a pretty harrowing ordeal, to say the least, although for the bovine boys I'm sure it was an adventure.

No strangers to multitasking, our first official fund-raiser was also Doug's and my wedding! It was a housewarming, farm-warming, organization-warming, and nuptials wrapped into one, and it was incredible. Of course we wanted to have the wedding at our new home. Since we were both enthusiastic cooks, we already had all the usual wedding-gift items—you know, the serving bowls and blenders—so we asked our 120 guests for donations toward the sanctuary instead.

Lord knows how we managed to organize a wedding while we were building the physical sanctuary and the organization, but it came off beautifully. Our outdoor ceremony was set against the fall-colored mountains surrounding our fields. Guests sat on hay bales while a bluegrass quartet played softly. Nearby in the pasture, Andy, Ralphie, and Elvis looked on with interest, and we could hear our hens clucking from beyond the reception tent. It was some blissful afternoon in that meadow, celebrating our mutual adoration with our beloved humans and animals. I could see my friends and family smile from their straw perches as I walked the grass aisle, holding a bouquet of wildflowers that Dan and Ashley had picked on our property that morning. I could see Doug, handsome in his suit, waiting for me. I could see our dear friend Kirsti set to officiate, ready to make us laugh all the way through.

During the ceremony, we read excerpts of e-mails from our

early long-distance courtship—some goofy, some romantic, some just a little raunchy. Kirsti, also a recording artist and angel-voiced singer, graced us with a stripped-down and slowed-down version of Robert Plant's "Sea of Love," Cat Power style, at my request. We finished up by reciting the lyrics to the *Green Acres* theme song in a mock Beat-poet style. All of us were cracking up. Then Doug and I lifted the back flap of the wedding tent to reveal a red vintage lawn tractor, hopped on, and rode right down the aisle.

Of course, our ceremony wasn't devoid of hints of our value system. After we exchanged vows, my friend Petrina from my TV production days read a powerful essay by John Robbins about humans' dynamic with farmed animals. I can still hear her deliver his powerful words as I fought back tears (like a total goober):

> When each of us comes to the end of our lives, what will matter is not what our social standing was, or whether the world thought we were important or influential. What will matter, what in fact always matters, are *the values we uphold and the principles and possibilities we stand for.* What will matter then, and what matters now, are the quality of the love we share with the world and the statements we make with our choices and our lives.

During the reception, Dan, a nationally syndicated cartoonist who also happens to be a stand-up comedian, sang a hilarious song he'd written about our wedding day, and made fun of my gorgeous and groovy tie-dyed wedding dress. He "played" a ridiculous cardboard cutout guitar. Susie stood up to speak, too. After laughing about times we shared together at Farm Sanctuary and our gross-out antics, she talked about the important role animal sanctuaries serve and her faith in us creating a magical and important place.

Meanwhile, the wine flowed and we chowed down. We'd hired a local vegan-friendly restaurant to cater the event. They served our favorite entrée there: blue-corn crusted seitan cutlets with chimichurri sauce, along with a full Southern vegan menu and a decadent chocolate wedding cake. After we'd stuffed ourselves, we encouraged guests to take the table decorations—miniature alfalfa bales—and feed them to the cows so they could stuff themselves, too, much to the delight of both humans and bovines.

Though neither of us have deep pockets in our families, our good-hearted friends and family helped us raise enough to finish acres of fencing and buy farm supplies. We couldn't have asked for anything better—and just in time.

Right after our wedding, Susie called. She'd been contacted by Wilderness Ranch, a well-established farm animal sanctuary in Loveland, Colorado. It was closing, and the sanctuary staff was reaching out to find homes or other sanctuaries that could take some of their more-difficult-to-place animals, like full-grown pigs. Farm Sanctuary was at capacity with pigs, and Susie wondered if we could help. We, of course, had room for them but no barn to shelter them . . . yet. We would need help—our operation was still too young for us to come up with the major bucks ($28,000) it would take to erect a barn and connect electricity and running water. Fortunately, Wilderness Ranch was able to work with their supporters and raise most of the funds. And through our efforts at fund-raising and soliciting volunteers, we got it built with an all-volunteer crew. We worked night and day for weeks to prepare to welcome the twelve well-socialized, 700-to-1,000-pound pigs, and the anticipation was killing me! Chris Kerr once again brought us his voluminous planning and construction talents and headed the team. Another friend, Mike Radzvilowicz, who'd once run a fowl sanctuary of his own, moved in with us for several months and volunteered all day every day to help build and set up.

Ten pigs from the group had started life out west at a crowded farm before they were purchased by a local brewery. The brewery owner wanted to use the piglets for the spectacle of "pig races" and then have a nice, festive pig roast at their end-of-summer festival. Wilderness Ranch stepped in and pleaded for the piglets' lives, even screening footage of pigs in factory farms. The brewery owner watched the pigs' jam-packed, deeply stressful trip to the slaughterhouse—which can often mean days without food and water in a constant state of sheer panic—and then, of course, their horror-show deaths. The video affected him enough to agree to give the pigs to the sanctuary—but only after the races.

The pigs were well cared for and loved for six years at Wilderness Ranch, and the thankful directors were relieved to find a new home where this older, bonded group could stay together and continue to live out their lives in peace. We sent the directors photos and videos of the progress of the barn and made plans to get the pigs to Woodstock. Their safe and legal transportation from Colorado was no small task. They had to undergo testing, a series of vaccinations, and painful piercings in their thick, sensitive ears to accommodate the tags they were forced to wear for interstate transportation.

The Lucky Ones

Finally, we welcomed Julie, Pig-Pig, Sophie, Dharma, Dolly, Louie, Stubby, Cromwell, Lodo, Zack, Wilbur, and Oliver. The transport trailer arrived on a miserably gray and sleety winter day with more than a foot of snow on the ground. We could hear snorts and grunts as the truck backed up to a side entrance of our new barn. Each of the pigs eagerly walked off the trailer, right into their cozy yet spacious straw-filled barn, to check out the new digs, and then made a beeline to the feed bowls in the pasture that awaited them. It was only after they snarfed down their meal of apples, potatoes, carrots, and overripe bananas (we wanted to make an impression) that they sauntered over to sniff us and acknowledge that we were even there. Then, without even checking out the rest of their pasture, they settled down in the barn and arranged themselves into their habitual groups and pairs. Beyond delighted, we went around to each pig, scratching ears and offering belly rubs—the receipt of which is their favorite activity besides eating.

I couldn't believe how quickly we were getting the sanctuary up and running. The first fifteen months were a whirlwind. I never imagined we would have gotten to where we were so quickly, and I was thankful for the opportunities that had arrived at our doorstep—literally, but I knew in order to continue to feed and care for all of our new animals we needed to open our doors to the public and begin really building our support base.

When you start a sanctuary, you imagine yourself feeding pigs, hugging cows, and scooping chicken poop, but alas, the reality involves as much paperwork, research, phone calls, applications, and number-crunching as any business. Contrary to the spelling of the word, there's no fun in fund-raising, but of course no organization succeeds without it. We had to figure out money before anything; we knew we couldn't be safe guardians to our animals without steady funding sources.

We started with our community. I introduced myself around town and set up a table in front of the local health food market, talking to passersby about our mission and work and signing up supporters and volunteers. We brought the table to festivals and fairs as well as to conferences and various other community gatherings. We contacted local media and New York City rescue groups. Then we began researching foundations that care about animals. And we set up a website and sent word to people we knew in the animal rescue and rights world, asking them to share our information with friends and to sign up for our new, online "e-Moosletter" where we would feature rescues, share important issues affecting farmed animals, and accept donations. Slowly but surely, we began to build a mailing list and a good-size group of supporters.

Finally, in 2006, when our ducks were in a row (or in this case, chickens, pigs, and cows—ducks came later), we threw open our barn doors to the public. By that time, we had nonprofit status and community support from people and institutions, elements we wanted before our official opening. We also had two full chicken coops, the three steer and twelve pigs, our Three Wise Men turkeys, and good old Olivia the goat.

We'd done a lot of PR for our grand-opening weekend, from radio interviews to ads in local papers to tabling, but I was terrified that no one would show. I was anxious until the last minute, and Doug had to calm me down (a fairly common pattern in our family). But thank goodness, I couldn't have been more wrong. Strangers piled out of their cars from all over the region to see what this new place was about, and friends, volunteers, and backers came to show their support on our big day. There were babies and toddlers and teens and adults and octogenarians. There was a middle-aged couple in matching sweatshirts that read VEGAN and a young guy in a camouflage hunting cap. There were kids in jeans and women in sundresses and sandals that they'd probably be sorry they'd worn by the end of the day. Car after car parked and unloaded.

I took groups of roughly a dozen people at a time around the farm and introduced them to almost each and every resident (those were the days when we had few enough residents to do that). I told them the animals' names, where they'd come from, and a little about their personalities, and then I talked about how billions like them live on today's farms. This was my first time talking directly to the public about issues concerning farm animals, so I was more than a little nervous. I had to keep honing my skills in those early days, figuring out based on the group whether I was coming on too strong, but most people seemed genuinely curious to learn about animals and our broken, cruel food system. I felt inspired by what I was getting from them, too: that more and more people were concerned about the welfare of animals, including farm animals.

Questions came at me from every side, and, much to my relief, I was able to answer ninety-nine percent of them. All my reading, research, animal care, and work at Farm Sanctuary paid off. There were plenty of facts-and-figures questions, and then some based on observation: "I never knew pigs could get so big! How much do those pigs weigh?" (Up to a thousand pounds!) "Why is that chicken on top of that other chicken?" (They're getting it on!) "Do those pigs bite? Are they mean? I've heard pigs have killed and eaten people!" (If they are stressed, crowded, starving, or mistreated, so have dogs, but not our happy pigs!)

After three years of thinking and training and planning and building, here I was face-to-face with people who had come to interact with these animals: to touch them and pet them and ask questions about them. This was one of only a handful of places in the country where people could look unexploited farm animals in the eye, and it was powerful and moving to watch people relate to them. Epiphanies, sadness, wonder, insight, surprise, apprehension—every visiting day, the blend of complicated emotions bowled me over. I saw anguish when people understood for the first time *who* they were eating. I saw relief to be among others who shared their values. I saw tears of joy from people delighted to watch these animals be themselves, which is an utterly beautiful thing. All of that happens here, and that is how change happens.

It's hard to believe that was five years ago. They have been some of the busiest, most challenging years of my life; they have also been the most rewarding. Since then, we have erected another large barn for the goats, sheep, and rabbits; built a duck and goose shed and installed a beautiful pond for them; constructed a building to house our visitors' center, offices, and medical treatment room, including an infirmary; built more coops; and erected more sheds for equipment storage. Finally, with the help of a very generous donor, we purchased an adjacent property with a 150-year-old house and barn that we've renovated into a bed and breakfast and intern housing. Whew!

We've also been really fortunate to have gained celebrity

support, which has helped the visibility of our mission and organization, something nonprofits can never get enough of. Luminaries such as Alicia Silverstone, Moby, Nigel Barker, Jim James, Sean Lennon, Chrissie Hynde, and Nellie McKay have come to visit and support our work, along with the band Mercury Rev, whose lead singer, Jonathan Donahue (formerly of the Flaming Lips), lives locally and is a friend and supporter. It's an indication of the growing understanding of farm animal issues in popular culture.

Animal lover Alicia Silverstone came early in our building process, and she and her husband had a great time lovin' on the animals, watching the construction of our goat and sheep barn, and snacking in our kitchen. Nellie McKay and Moby came by near the beginning, too; they'd both heard about us through mutual friends Dan and Ashley. But the other musicians came by more circuitous means.

A couple of years ago, my sister and I went to Louisville for a family visit, and we decided to grab a bite at a favorite restaurant. I glanced around and noticed Jim James, lead singer of the popular band My Morning Jacket, sitting at the table right next to us. I was a little starstruck. The band had sold out Madison Square Garden the prior New Year's Eve, and I had been disappointed that I couldn't go. I knew Jim and the band were based in Louisville, but I never expected to run into them. Though I snuck plenty of looks at him (and at his plate—his meal was vegan!) and started a few conversations in my head, I didn't approach him. I kicked myself for that more than once when I got home.

But the very next day, out again at a different restaurant with my mother, who walked in but Jim James! We gave each other a look of recognition, and this time I resolved to say hello. I ordered a beer as liquid courage, and headed over just as he was leaving.

"Hey," I started. "I'm a fan and a native Louisvillian. And I don't know if you're a supporter of animal causes, but I run a farmed animal sanctuary and I couldn't help but notice that yesterday and today you seem to be eating meatless meals." I told him about the sanctuary and our mission, and invited him to come up anytime he found himself in New York. And could I be so bold as to ask if he would ever consider performing at a benefit concert, like our friends Nellie McKay and Mercury Rev had in the recent past? He was so warm and supportive and genuinely enthusiastic about our work. Turned out that my hunch about his diet was right—well almost, I think he's a pescetarian (he still eats fish). He was also proud that another Louisvillian had gone off to do something good in the world. He is often quoted talking about his love of Louisville and the kind of people it breeds. I asked him if we could be in touch and gave him my card. He then, surprisingly, scribbled his e-mail down and said he looked forward to talking more.

I have to say I thought there was a chance he might have put on a show to be nice and given me a false address. Fortunately, that wasn't the case, and we corresponded during the months that followed. He is genuinely a super-nice guy. While he was too busy with his new album to do a benefit concert right away, he had another idea. He decided to release an EP, a tribute to George Harrison, under his moniker Yim Yames, and he wanted proceeds to go to us. He wrote me that he'd heard George was "always about treating all creatures equally and eating responsibly, so it just made sense" to support us through the EP. I was floored. On the front of every vinyl album and CD is a big gold sticker that says, "A portion of the proceeds of this album goes to Woodstock Farm Animal Sanctuary" and includes our Web address. Not only was it a generous and beautiful gesture, it also brought a major increase in awareness about our sanctuary—and much-needed and much-appreciated funds!

When I heard about the EP, I called Fernanda Santos, who'd written the piece on Albie for *The New York Times*, brimming over. "Think you might be able to help us get some good press on this besides album reviews?" I asked her.

"Let me run it by the music editor," she said. She ended up interviewing Jim and me AND George Harrison's widow. She covered everything—our chance meeting, the new EP, the work and mission of WFAS. It was a great story that brought in even more attention to our work and our mission. And it led to another score: after he read the article, Jason Fine, the executive editor of *Rolling Stone*, called me up. He and his wife, musician Tracy Bonham, had a place in Woodstock and were dying to come check us out. We became fast friends, and Jason, with his many connections, wanted to help us raise some money and thought having concerts at the farm would be a cool way to do so. He connected us to Chrissie Hynde and Sean Lennon, both of whom performed sold-out benefit concerts at the farm, raising more funds for the sanctuary.

Chrissie Hynde posed for pictures before her concert, and she especially loved holding Rod the rooster, who turned into a pile of goo in her arms. Sean Lennon sang with his partner Charlotte Kemp Muhl, who lay down and snuggled with two pigs for a photo op. Doug captioned the resulting picture, "Judy and Patsy complained later that Charlotte made them look fat in this photo." Sean posed with Fern the goat, both with serious faces. A week later, Sean wrote us that his gig at the farm was "one of the most pleasant experiences I've ever had on the road, and I've had a few, believe me." He also said being at the sanctuary made him and Charlotte "wonder how we can be better model citizens for animal rights." (That's what an afternoon with Patsy and Judy can do to you.) They offered to continue helping us out and visiting when they could, and they came again just a week later for more animal time and photos, and enjoyed eating at the great vegan restaurant in town, the Garden Cafe on the Green.

I asked Sean—once again, my shamelessness at play—if he could get a letter from me to Paul McCartney. He did, and within a week, I turned on my computer and almost had a heart attack. There in my e-mail in-box, a subject line read, "Note from Paul McCartney." Wha?!?! He wrote that he had heard about us from Sean and was pleased to hear about the work we did. He also said he'd heard great things about us from Chrissie. That's right, folks, Paul McCartney e-mailed me. And it was arranged by our mutual friend Sean Lennon. And he had a conversation with Chrissie Hynde about us. I had to be scraped off the floor. Doug and I high-fived each other so many times that day that my hand was sore by dinnertime.

10

Soapbox Feet

My husband once called me "the girl who was born with soapboxes instead of feet." I'm not shy about expressing my opinions, and my opinions are strong on certain topics, as you may have noticed. But I have learned the hard way that people don't want to be preached at; it's not a way to change hearts and minds. When I've got people on a tour—the "captive audience" I mentioned at the beginning of this book—I might appear from the outside to be simply telling some animal stories mixed with facts. But under the hood there's a whole mechanism at work. I'm reading their faces. Am I making eye contact? Should I let those distracted parents of the toddler off the hook and focus on these college kids instead? Am I going into too much detail? Will the vegan-tattooed punk guy think I'm lame if I don't talk about forced molting of egg-laying hens? Is it worth repeating some information for the couple that arrived late? Is that a raindrop I just felt?

Fortunately for me, you the reader are (hopefully) not distracted by a toddler, tattoos, latecomers, or rain, so I'd like to kick off my (my dogs are aching anyway) and dive into some ... The topic has gotten so big and broad there are now graduate degrees in Humane Education, Animal Policy and Law, Animal Rights Theory, to name a few, and there's lots to say. Here's "the gospel according to Jenny Brown," which includes some heavy lifting from the tremendously talented writers and activists who preceded me.

Eating is a political and social action. Environmental destruction, public health, workers' rights, decaying rural communities, world hunger, and global poverty are all deeply affected by our eating choices. Of course, when we're stuffing our gobs at the dinner table, eating beyond fullness and rushing through the meal, we're not going to stop to think about these issues, much less the plight of animals. We don't ask ourselves, "How did this animal live?" or "What did my dollars support by buying this?" Much less "Could I have killed this animal myself?" That would involve mindfulness that we are eating an animal in the first place. We rarely see who is raised for our food and don't have to witness their deaths, so it's easy to avoid thinking about eating animals at all. And we like it that way.

Our disassociation starts fairly early: Most children are naturally sympathetic to farm animals, but parents, teachers, and others, already indoctrinated into a society built on convenience and habit, distract children from the brutal realities of our food system. But do we really want to lie to our kids and discourage them from asking the important questions?

Whether we like it or not, today's consumers are responsible for the worst systematic animal abuse in world history. We can point fingers at the Big Bad Corporations—and I do—but this system is sustained by consumer demand. If we don't enable corporations to profit from suffering, they can't. It's incredibly empowering to take a stance that moves us all in that direction. As Jonathan Safran Foer has written, "One of the greatest opportunities to live our values—or betray them—lies in the food we put on our plates. And we will live or betray our values not only as individuals, but as nations."

At the very least, a person who chooses not to support farm animal exploitation is assured a clearer conscience. That person helps change the economy of animal farming. "Never doubt that a *small group* of thoughtful, committed citizens can change the world," Margaret Mead said. "Indeed, it is *the only thing that ever has*."

Those tiny calves destined for veal that I filmed back in Texas years ago, the ones born to dairy cows, are in every glass of milk and slice of cheese. Pigs are strung up by one foot while they are still flailing from a bolt shot into their brains, have their throats slit, feet cut off, and are skinned—sometimes while still conscious— for BLTs and pepperoni. The chicks in the garbage behind laying operations, and the laying hens who endure the most miserable life of any animal, are in every egg salad sandwich and jar of mayonnaise. Broiler hens are flipped upside down, shackled, and slashed with a blade, then plunged into scalding water, often while still alive, so that their bodies can become "healing, comforting" chicken noodle soup. The violence behind choices has been whitewashed to oblivion.

Melanie Joy, a psychologist and professor, talks about this disconnect in her book *Why We Love Dogs, Eat Pigs, and Wear Cows*. Many of our beliefs about eating animals, she says, are based on cultural or societal traditions that we don't question: "We don't need meat to survive or even be healthy; millions of healthy and long-lived vegetarians have proven this point. We eat animals simply because it's what we've always done, and because we like the way they taste. Most of us eat animals because it's just the way things are."

If those are indeed the best reasons we can come up with, Joy continues, then something's wrong: "What could cause an entire society of people to check their thinking caps at the door—*and to not even realize they're doing so?*" We can become prisoners of our earliest indoctrinations or we can choose to look critically at our assumptions and align our lives with our values. Choosing to live vegan is how we are able to do that best.

■ ■ ■ ■

Some people say, "Well, okay, I'll just avoid animal products from factory farms." Those farms are indeed the most egregious offenders, the greatest symbol of our dismaying disconnect from and disrespect for animals. And they are "home" to ninety-nine percent of U.S. farm animals. But whenever and wherever living beings' bodies are used to make a profit, animals suffer. And their unnecessary deaths are the ultimate injustice, no matter how "naturally" they are raised or "humanely" they are slaughtered. And isn't "humane slaughter" an oxymoron? While it's conceivable that a small "family" farmer with a few chickens in the yard or a cow in a barn would feel a respectful, symbiotic relationship with his or her animals, those animals still die in violent ways. Whether a knife to the throat or a shot in the head, it's violent. Make no mistake: There's nothing humane about it.

My years of farm animal rescue and advocacy have taught me that even small farms engage in cruel practices. The chicks used for eggs come from the same hatcheries where male chicks are thrown out with the trash and hens are killed once their production declines. Calves, lambs, and kids (baby goats) are torn from their mothers in order for humans to drink the milk. Castration, male culling (killing the males), branding, tail docking, dehorning, debeaking, debilling, toe and snood amputation: these are common practices at quaint "local" farms and large operations alike.

Since food labeling is so deeply problematic, we can't consider ourselves educated consumers if we simply trust the "free-range" or "cage-free" or "all-natural" stamp on the carton. These terms aren't regulated and can be false or extremely misleading. They reduce consumers' guilt, but we don't know unless we've monitored a farm's full process what really goes on, no matter how happy the illustrated hen or cow looks on the package or what the label claims. For instance, free range is supposed to dictate that animals have access to the outdoors. But that can mean a tiny area accessible through one narrow door for thousands, even tens of thousands, of animals who live the rest of their lives crowded into an indoor shed. Only the term "organic" is monitored, but it just means that the animals eat feed grown without pesticides, antibiotics, or hormones and are not injected with the latter two. It does *not* mean animals are treated humanely.

No, the only way to know for sure that you're not supporting cruelty is to avoid animal products altogether. It's like this: I'd like to think that if I had lived in pre–Civil War America, I would have been an outspoken abolitionist, and that, while I would probably have focused my activism on the most horrific plantations, I would have chosen to support no slave owners at all.

There's a word that gets in the way when people think about changing their diets: *comfortable*. We feel entitled to comfort, and that often means taking the path of least resistance: ultimate convenience. It's easy to be able to pull into any diner, or patronize a fast-food drive-thru, or sit down at anyone's table for dinner, or grab whatever's offered to you at a party without having to think about what you're eating or be a squeaky wheel. Those are natural, understandable impulses.

The thing is, once a person understands how animals are abused and slaughtered, can we be comfortable participating in this system? To me, supporting cruelty creates a far deeper discomfort. Even though being vegan does mean saying no when I'm offered a burger at a barbecue and sometimes means eating a baked potato and an iceberg-lettuce salad at some crappy roadside restaurant when you are starving, it also creates a sense of inner comfort that I find worth way more than occasionally eating a boring meal. If preventing suffering and death isn't worth sacrifice, what is?

That's another word I'd like to examine—sacrifice. When a third of the planet doesn't have enough to eat, and most people around the world eat the same thing almost every day, my fridge full of delicious and healthy options keeps me from feeling like I'm doing much sacrificing. The Western world, especially the United States, has an unequaled abundance and diversity of food. Is it really a sacrifice to limit ourselves to a great bounty of foods instead of an unlimited bounty of foods?

I've always been puzzled that people otherwise willing to question norms and think for themselves—people who seem really caring and compassionate, who profess their love for animals—have a blind spot when it comes to their role in keeping animal industries wealthy and widespread. There are so many artists, educators, activists, freethinkers, and just plain good people who will question many mandates and customs and work to understand issues—and shut their ears to this particular one.

Meanwhile, the meat, dairy, and egg industries have done a brilliant snow job on us. We've been told since we were tiny that bright-eyed Elsie the Cow is eager to feed our children her milk. Celebrities in glossy magazines tell us her milk is good for us. We've got a brand-new United States Department of Agriculture food "plate" (replacing the pyramid) that still specifically recommends dairy. A fat steak is a symbol of wealth and success. Chickens are to be consumed in quantities requiring a bucket, and all-you-can-eat shrimp is a popular Red Lobster favorite. The beef industry has just launched the Masters of Beef Advocacy program (!), an online course that teaches college students and others how to talk up meat through social media and school and community presentations. The pork industry has the charming (by which I mean grotesque) "Pork4Kids" website, propagandizing kids ages six through fifteen, offering games and activities, photos of farm kids with happy pigs, and a "fun food zone." Then there's the iconic campaigns pummeling us at every turn, like "Pork: The other white meat," and the hot-off-the-press "Pork: Be Inspired." Are you kidding? How about the classic "Beef: It's what's for dinner." (I had a great bumper sticker for years that tells the real story: "Beef: It's what's rotting in your colon.")

Is this whitewashing fair? I think it's dangerous. Consider the myth of the "naturalness" of animal products. I've heard repeatedly, for instance, that it's better to eat butter made from cows' milk than nondairy butter because it's more "natural." But the process of making butter strikes me as anything but natural. First, a worker "milks" the semen out of a bull—meaning he or she masturbates him. Then, the dairy farmer who purchased that semen pushes his arm up a cow's vagina to artificially inseminate her. A calf begins to grow, and eventually the cow's body begins to manufacture a food suited perfectly to that calf, food that will go through the calf's four stomachs and help him or her grow hundreds of pounds within a few months.

But instead of having her calf's mouth on them, the mother's teats are fitted with synthetic-lined metal cups. Her milk is sucked through tubes into a large vat. Because her teats are clamped repeatedly by a machine instead of the mouth they were designed for, she endures painful chafing and mastitis—an infection in her udder—which often leads to pus draining into the milk. Meanwhile, the cow has most likely been administered hormones and genetically manipulated so that she will produce up to ten times the amount of milk she would produce naturally. As a result, her body is under constant stress, and she is at risk for numerous health problems, which causes the farmer to add antibiotics to this "natural" cocktail. Then, instead of nourishing a newborn, that milk is taken to factories where it is separated, analyzed for fat content, pasteurized to destroy enzymes and microorganisms, sucked into an electric churn via a plate heat exchanger, separated again, and churned again. Sometimes iodized salt is added. Viola! "Natural" butter.

Humans are the only species that drinks milk beyond infancy. And humans are the only species that drinks the milk of another species. After umpteen steps and heavy processing, we humans turn it into various foods and call it natural. And we never stop to think about what it really is: the breast milk of a cow. BREAST MILK, PEOPLE! From a COW. The thought of drinking human breast milk or eating cheese made from it disgusts most people. But at least it would come from our own species (and from women who would actually have a say in the matter)—wouldn't that actually be more "natural"? Why don't we drink giraffe milk or cat milk or pig milk? Sound gross? What's the difference?

My friend Gretchen works as a professor and administrator in a prison college program. One of her students, Intel, is an ethical vegan, which is insanely hard to pull off in a prison environment. (Gretchen tells people, "If he can do it in there, there's no excuse for people not doing it out here!") Intel wrote an essay about his experience becoming vegan while incarcerated and published it in *American Vegan* magazine. He links becoming vegan to becoming more mature, going from reckless teen to responsible man. And he makes a connection between cruelty to animals and human violence, highlighting the desensitization that underlies both. "Learning of the environmental and moral implications of an animal-free diet helped foster my growing empathy for people I had hurt," he writes. "I became a man determined to reclaim his humanity by embracing all life."

I believe that there are ways in which Intel, a vegan man who puts on a prison uniform each morning, has more freedom than most Americans. As my friend and fellow animal activist Sharon Gannon teaches, "How can we ourselves hope to be free and happy when our lives are rooted in depriving others of the very thing we say we value most in life—the freedom to pursue happiness?"

Isaac Bashevis Singer, the great Nobel Prize–winning Yiddish writer and a staunch vegetarian, also connected human and animal violence when he wrote, "When a human kills an animal for food, he is neglecting his own hunger for justice. Man prays for mercy, but is unwilling to extend it to others.... It is inconsistent."

Echoes of those parallels run through the comparison that many philosophers, writers, and activists make between Nazi Germany and today's factory farms. Singer, who escaped Poland but who lost much of his family, community, and culture to the Nazis, made the connection between the Holocaust and mass animal slaughter many times in his books and interviews. In his short story "The Letter Writer," he refers to farm animals as enduring "an eternal Treblinka." This is a controversial stance. I along with many others agree with Singer. He argues that human beings see oppression clearly when *we* are the victims. Otherwise we victimize blindly and thoughtlessly.

Charles Patterson, a Holocaust educator who came to animal issues later in his career, was so influenced by Singer that he called his book *Eternal Treblinka*. Patterson relates the roots of the Holocaust to "the human arrogance behind animal exploitation and the vast array of injustices against humans which have flowed from it." Many believe that examining this analogy trivializes the Holocaust, but Patterson disagrees: "The claim that the exploitation and destruction of the other inhabitants of the earth is 'trivial' says a lot about the person making such a claim." Patterson was also influenced by the late animal and AIDS activist Steven Simmons, who argued that animals are victims of a system that believes some lives are more valuable than others and that those with power can do what they wish to the powerless.

When we actually think about animals' capacity to suffer, is it really fair to draw such a deep line between our species that we ridicule people who are saddened and appalled by deliberate cruelty to animals *and* humans alike?

Choosing a vegan diet connects us to the food we eat. It says we are aware of the processes that bring food to our plates. That we feel living beings have been given the gift of consciousness and that life is precious to each of us. It's a realization that life is not ours to take, especially when life is taken simply to satisfy our taste buds. It says we want a kinder, healthier society. This is something that benefits humans and animals alike in so many ways, which is why I'm often puzzled when people question the worth of concentrating on animals—as if human and animal interests were somehow mutually exclusive.

The first step to changing your outlook and diet is to get educated. We live in the Information Age: In no other time has it been easier, nor more vital, to be a conscious consumer. Try perusing a few of the many books and articles on the subject, or Googling simple phrases like "Why vegan?" YouTube has a host of undercover videos that show us the grisly realities of modern-day animal factories and slaughter. For better or worse, a YouTube search for "farm animal abuse" will inspire you to take steps against what you see. And what you see will outrage you. It can be very difficult to watch, but for justice to prevail, we need to be outraged. *We must not refuse to see with our eyes what they must endure with their bodies.*

Part of the problem is that the mainstream media doesn't show these images and rarely touches upon farm animal issues. It's too unpleasant and uncomfortable, and networks fear they could lose valuable advertisers (corporate food chains, meat and dairy products) if programs examine the realities of animal agriculture. I don't mean to make journalists the bad guys here, but with enormous human health and safety, financial, and animal welfare issues in the balance, why aren't we being told more?

There's so much to learn, even beyond the deep ethical concerns. So many myths understandably swirl around our dinner tables. But people can easily get enough protein. Meat isn't as natural for us as we've been told—the human body's better suited to a vegetarian diet. And longevity of practice sure isn't a good excuse. As Isaac Bashevis Singer said, "People often say that humans have always eaten animals, as if this is a justification for continuing the practice. According to this logic, we should not try to prevent people from murdering other people, since this has also been done since the earliest of times."

Some people ask, "But what would happen to all the animals if we stopped eating them? Won't they become extinct or be set loose and cause mayhem?" This is almost as silly as people asking if my foot is real when I mention my fake leg (this happens more often than you'd think). Industries must respond to consumer demand in order to remain profitable, so if demand for eggs, meat, and milk gradually decreased, fewer and fewer animals would be raised for food. Nearly all farm animals are artificially bred, and bred repeatedly for as often and as long as possible. Left to their own devices, animals would not reproduce anywhere near as much.

So not only does choosing a plant-based diet save animal lives, it leads farmers to turn to healthier, more environmentally friendly agriculture. This means the price of organic produce goes down and our quality of life goes up. Eventually, if the pattern continues, the only farm animals around will be beloved, respected companion animals living healthy lives. At least this is the dream.

Cutting down on animal products is a wonderful step along the path to conscious eating. Less is less: Eating fewer animal products means less demand for them. As you familiarize yourself with delicious alternatives and great veg restaurants, you'll probably want to make more changes. You can reduce consumption simply by choosing a day of the week to eat vegetarian; a project called Meatless Monday can help on that score. Or you can begin substituting vegan products for certain staples (check out some of my favorites at the end of the book). Trust me—once you try Purely Decadent's Mocha Almond Fudge coconut milk ice cream, you won't want to go back to Edy's.

Are you a homebody? You can also try armchair activism: helping animals from the comfort of your home by just sitting down to a keyboard or picking up the phone. Write elected officials and newspapers about animal protection bills and the negative impacts of animal farming. Voice your support for vegan options in restaurants, school cafeterias, university dining halls, or workplace eateries. Vegan food has found its way into schools, airports, and workplaces thanks to public pressure. (Amtrak recently started offering a veggie burger, which means now vegans can have a horrible meal on a train just like everyone else!) Proposition 2 in California, a ballot initiative that prohibits some of the worst abuses suffered by egg-laying chickens, pregnant sows, and veal calves, passed in a landslide as a direct result of grassroots organizing, public support, and the members of organizations like Farm Sanctuary; the Humane Society of the United States; Physicians Committee for Responsible Medicine (PCRM); and other animal welfare, environmental, and religious organizations. Meanwhile, PETA members have done a great job pressuring companies to stop testing products on animals and urging farms, restaurants, high school science labs, and circuses to drop the cruelty.

We can also change the world by fighting against the drastically skewed subsidies for meat and dairy. How in the world can a Big Mac cost less than a head of broccoli?! The answer is—well, corruption. The power of the meat and dairy lobbies is *staggering*. According to a PCRM study, seventy-four percent of our federal subsidies go to meat and dairy, even though—now here's some irony for you—federal nutrition recommendations feature grains, vegetables, and fruits as far more paramount to a healthy diet! Why? The Center for Science in the Public Interest, a consumer advocacy organization, tells us:

> The answers . . . are matters of politics, not science, and typically revolve around money and livelihoods. The makers of pesticides, fertilizer, and animal drugs; the cattle, hog, poultry, and dairy industries; the large grain companies and grain farmers—they all defend the status quo. They pour millions of dollars each year into campaign contributions, lobbyists' salaries, and advertising campaigns. They wine and dine politicians— often over fatty steaks—and use hardball tactics to rein in any rare elected official who dares stray from the proper path. . . . And, by making use of the "revolving door," top officials from the cattle, pork, dairy, and other food- and agriculture-related industries become top officials in the U.S. Department of Agriculture, and many former legislators and Department of Agriculture officials enjoy more lucrative, and no less influential, careers on Washington's K Street, where they lobby for those industries.

The *New York Times* food writer Mark Bittman bemoans this state of affairs. "Imagine [farm subsidies] designed to encourage a resurgence of small- and medium-size farms producing not corn syrup and animal-feed but food we can touch, see, buy and eat—like apples and carrots—while diminishing handouts to agribusiness and its political cronies," he writes. He suggests diverting funds from the foods that make us obese and ruin our environment—the animal food crops and the animal food itself—and using that money to pay farmers who grow fruits, veggies, and beans; to research sustainable agriculture; and to recruit new small farmers. Bittman wants subsidies to do what they are intended to: "encourage the development of the kind of agriculture we need, one that prioritizes caring for the land, the people who work it and the people who need the real food that's grown on it."

And that's a lot of people. There's a lot of talk about food security around the world, but we have plenty of food for everyone as long as we're not diverting appalling amounts of land and water to grow animal feed and raise livestock. According to EarthSave International, cattle consume a whopping seventy percent of U.S. grain. For every sixteen pounds of grain fed to a beef cow, we get only one pound of edible flesh back. (The other fifteen pounds are used by the animal to produce energy or to make some part of its own body that we don't eat, like blood, bones, skin, or hair, or it is excreted.) And water? It takes 2,500 gallons of it to produce that one pound of beef. The same amount could grow more than fifty pounds of fruits and vegetables.

If you consider the feeding, housing, transporting, and slaughtering of animals, and then the packing and transporting of the flesh and products themselves, you're looking at tremendous exploitation and degradation of natural resources. Producing a calorie of meat protein means burning more than ten times as much fossil fuel—and spewing more than ten times as much heat-trapping carbon dioxide—as does a calorie of plant protein.

Since ten times the land needed to grow flora for human consumption is needed to grow plants for livestock, land is in great demand. The result means destroying great swaths of rainforest and other wilderness. More than sixty percent of the Amazon rainforest, in fact, is now used for grazing pastures for cattle. According to University of Maryland professor emeritus Steve Boyan, "Every second of every day, one football field of tropical rainforest is destroyed in order to produce 257 hamburgers." This in turn leads to the endangerment and extinction of countless species. According to EarthSave, "For every pound of rainforest beef, approximately 650 pounds of precious living matter is destroyed, including 20–30 different plant species, over 100 insect species, and dozens of birds, mammals, and reptiles." And consider the people who rely on a symbiotic relationship with the forest. Is our beef habit more important than their lives? Consider also that the world's necessary oxygen filter is being destroyed, jeopardizing air quality. And that the burning of these forests means the expulsion of all the toxins and carbon dioxide these trees filter, an awful blow to our atmosphere.

The bottom line on this issue is that caring about the environment means more than recycling or turning down the heat in the winter or driving a fuel-efficient car. It means changing the way we eat. A recent United Nations report on livestock and the environment could hardly be more sobering: The livestock sector emerges as one of the top two or three most significant contributors to the most serious environmental problems, at every scale from local to global.

As for health, study after study has shown that animal products are unnecessary for a healthy diet and often stand in the way of one. Just a few of the respected organizations and journals that have reported on the health benefits of vegan diets are the American Cancer Society, Harvard University School of Public Health, the Physicians Committee for Responsible Medicine, *The American Journal of Clinical Nutrition*, the *American Journal of Epidemiology*, *Preventive Medicine*, *Pediatrics*, the *American Journal of Public Health*, and the *British Medical Journal* (*BMJ*). Even the Academy of Nutrition and Dietetics has declared vegan diets not only healthful and nutritionally adequate in every life stage, but also beneficial to—read, *superior* to—the Standard American Diet in the prevention and treatment of many diseases. We have been lied to our entire lives, and it's time to dispel the myth that animal-based foods are healthy.

Two doctors, T. Colin Campbell and Caldwell Esselstyn, have spent decades working to do just that: show the medical field and consumers just how *un*healthy and *un*necessary animal products are. Dr. Campbell's groundbreaking work *The China Study* exhaustively details what happened to the health of Chinese people when they began adopting a Western, flesh-based diet. The results, which involved research by Cornell University, Oxford University, and the Chinese Academy of Preventive Medicine, are chilling and clear: People who ate the most animal-based foods suffered the most chronic disease, and those who ate the most plant-based foods were the healthiest and tended to avoid chronic disease. The research also found that, amazingly enough, dairy actually weakens bones. Contrary to what the dairy industry has been hammering into us for generations, animal protein is highly acidic, so it leaches calcium from bones and expels it from the body. In fact, countries with the highest consumption of dairy have the highest incidence of osteoporosis.

In all, Campbell meticulously lays out the evidence for more than 8,000 statistically relevant correlations between diet and disease. The good news is that he also shows that heart disease, diabetes, and obesity can be reversed by a healthy vegan diet.

Dr. Caldwell Esselstyn's twenty-year study of heart disease came to a similar conclusion. His work, which was presented in his book *Prevent and Reverse Heart Disease*, proved that switching to a low-fat, plant-based diet can not only prevent and stop the progression of heart disease, but also reverse its course. Heart disease is the leading killer in Western civilization and costs the United States alone more than $250 *billion* a year. Shouldn't we be preventing it and finding healthy remedies instead of scrambling for expensive, invasive surgical stopgap measures and pharmaceuticals? Dr. Esselstyn has had overwhelming and unequivocal success transitioning patients from what he calls "the toxic American diet" to a healthy vegan diet.

These two doctors, along with many others, make it plain: Eating animal products puts us at greater risk for stroke, diabetes, heart disease, obesity, osteoporosis, and several types of cancer such as colon and hormone-related cancers. The way to stay healthy is to stay away from animal products.

If animal foods aren't necessary or even healthy, continuing to eat meat, dairy, and eggs is only a nod to our palates and ingrained habits. And palates and habits just aren't good reasons to continue a horror show of a food system.

Gene Baur sums up many of these issues beautifully when he

says, "Instead of turning swords into ploughshares, the industrialization of agriculture has resulted in violence, corruption, cruelty, and pollution, and we ingest it at every meal." Delicious vegan food choices are a way to counter that, and in doing so, pursue justice. It feels empowering to fight the good fight just by making compassionate choices at the table. When most people are honest with themselves, I believe they feel the same. I think once they understand what's going on, most people would rather please their palates with kind foods, form more humane habits, and choose compassion over killing.

The Happy Endings

Apart of the sanctuary was sick. Olivia, our very first goat, was such an important part of the farm that it was hard to imagine the place without her. A proud member of the Free-Roamers—animals like the turkeys and certain chickens not assigned to a specific yard—she was an ever-present soul overseeing all the action at the farm.

"It's lymphoma," said our faithful vet, Dr. Rosenberg. He looked at Olivia's recent weight loss and blood work and gave her only a few months to live. We notified our staff, volunteers, and her legions of fans that Olivia's time was limited. The response was tremendous: If she was treated like a queen before, now she was treated like a queen on steroids. Speaking of steroids, they wouldn't help her, but we did research for alternative treatments. A friend steered us toward something called Hoxsey tonic. The story goes that a chap named Hoxsey observed a dramatic change in the eating habits of a horse with cancer; he isolated the types of leaves and herbs the horse was eating and, essentially, bottled them. We figured it certainly couldn't hurt, and Olivia loved the taste of the sweet elixir.

Perhaps it helped. Her spirit remained strong as fall crept into winter. However, when we got hit by the first Catskills snowstorm and a bitter chill came in the air, Olivia started having trouble standing up. One of our caregivers, Amber Plaut, noticed that she was shivering in her pen despite her insulated coat and blankets over her. At the time, our animal rehabilitation building was still in the fund-raising stages, so Doug and I made an executive decision: We would take her to live in our house, so that her final days would at least be comfortable. Doug created a pen just inside our back door, lined it with old sheets and straw, and used a plastic toboggan to transport Olivia over the bumpy snowbanks to her new, makeshift hospice.

Once settled in, she perked up. She essentially was in a corner of our large kitchen, where there's lots of action, and this was endlessly entertaining for her. Getting to see *where* the snacks came from and having close interactions with the house dogs and cats were new experiences for Olivia, and she seemed to be reveling in it all. The UPS guy did a double take the first time he knocked on the door and a goat responded. So what if around dinnertime our kitchen smelled of sautéed garlic and goat urine? She was happy, and so were we.

One day a friend stopped by who knows a thing or two about cancer herself. Kris Carr has been battling a rare and incurable stage-four cancer and is an expert on wellness. She suggested that we buy Olivia some wheatgrass and told us more than we knew about its many benefits. People pay good money for tiny shots made of the stuff, and goats certainly like grass, so wasn't it worth a try?

The Happy Endings

We bought a tray from the local health food place (not cheap—it's $20 a tray) and set it in front of her. It was gone within minutes, and we were on the phone looking to score wheatgrass at wholesale prices.

You can see where this is leading: We had a goat as a roommate for the entire winter. This was on top of the usual menagerie of sick chickens and other critters stacked in cages at the opposite end of the house. Our appliance repairman was called more than once to address issues with the washing machine—constantly running poopy towels and sheets through it took a toll.

When the weather warmed up, Olivia went back to her usual spot in the pig barn. I'm so proud that she continued to have an excellent quality of life for many more months, beating our vet's estimate by nearly a year. After she died, a group of admirers collected, and we scattered her ashes in a shady spot she had enjoyed on hot summer days.

Our urine-soaked subfloor might disagree, but I would do it all over again if I had to. Fortunately, we now have a building dedicated to this purpose, and the smell in the kitchen has faded away, but our memory of Olivia and her incredible story will never go away. Her complex personality taught us so much about animals and people and what they mean to each other.

I often envision a giant protective bubble over our property, and inside it a place where everything is right in the world, the way we want it to be. Animals roam free, living happy and peaceful lives the way they should. They are free to be themselves, among friends and, in some cases, family. There is no more fear of harm, no want for food or water, warmth or shelter. They have everything they need. They are loved, and treated with respect and compassion, until their dying moments in our arms, when they are wet from our tears. We coexist with them, never considering ourselves superior or their "owners." We don't use them as commodities or exploit them in any way. They are our friends. Beloved friends. They owe us nothing. But what they do give, unconsciously, is the greatest asset to our work. They are ambassadors for all others like them, showing humans that other animals are not mere automatons.

■ ■ ■ ■

Visitors to Woodstock Farm Animal Sanctuary bear witness to the scars left by industrial confinement, cruel handling and procedures, and the long-term effects of breeding for productivity. They can see and touch the battery cages, farrowing crate (for pregnant pigs), and veal crate that we have on display for educational purposes. Visitors also bear witness to the love and care we provide to these animals as our staff caretakers and volunteers perform physical therapy, administer medications, and provide special diets to special needs animals all around the farm, on top of cleaning their barns and sheds all day every day. We work our tails off, providing the best care possible to every animal who comes through our doors. It's a top priority to us, although incredibly expensive, time-consuming, and often heartbreaking. But it's an obligation we have to them and a profound responsibility.

But I don't mean to make it all sound depressing and serious, because there is a tremendous amount of joy here, too—for the animals *and* the people. This is a sanctuary for humans as well. It's a happy-ending place where animals are given a second chance.

And it's a safe place where people are allowed to let their guard down and be with others who feel the way they do about animals. Many visit often just to spend time with the animals they have gotten to know and grown to love. Others who volunteer feel good about being a part of the work we're doing and for our cause in general.

I certainly can't take credit for all this. WFAS is much bigger than Doug, me, and our hardworking team. From the beginning, people have come out of the woodwork to do, well, woodwork: building barns, constructing fences, helping with rescues and fund-raisers. Just the reward they get from helping our fellow creatures draws wonderful people to us. The very idea of what we're doing has led many to offer their time, skills, energy, and financial support for Woodstock Farm Animal Sanctuary. The love and support that created a refuge for the most ignored, exploited, and mistreated animals on earth constitute the foundation on which WFAS was built. It has taken a small army, hundreds of thousands of dollars, and seven years to get to where we are today. None of it has been easy, but no one said it would be. In fact, some said explicitly that it wouldn't be. The reward for us is the love and appreciation the animals show us every day and witnessing the growing number of people who not only care but also are changing their dietary habits and adopting a more conscious and compassionate lifestyle. Together we are all, as Gandhi said, "being the change we want to see in the world."

There is also growing hope arising outside our little bubble. Media are finally beginning to give voice to some of the most egregious issues concerning factory farming. There have been major articles in top newspapers across the country, and exposés like

Death on a Factory Farm on HBO; and television producers and hosts like Ellen DeGeneres, Oprah Winfrey, and CNN's Jane Velez-Mitchell invite guests (like me!) to speak about our society's systematic abuse of farmed animals and the implications on our health and environment. (Velez-Mitchell, who is vegan, recently had me promote a compassionate ThanksLiving event that we hold every year at the sanctuary.) This is brave territory for them (though Oprah could be braver). Also, vegan and vegetarian restaurants are popping up all over the place, and healthy vegan fast-food businesses, like Blossom Du Jour in New York City, are becoming popular. Vegan food carts are making their way into urban and not-so-urban areas across the country, and everywhere you look, vegetarian and vegan items are continually being added to menus to meet growing demand. Healthy and delicious meat and dairy alternatives like Field Roast, Tofurky, Vegenaise, and Daiya Cheese are also appearing in grocery stores around the country, and grocery chains like Trader Joe's and Whole Foods carry a great selection of vegan items and meat and dairy substitutes. There are more animal advocacy organizations than ever before, and sanctuaries like ours are growing in numbers, too.

Jonathan Safran Foer's *Eating Animals* includes one of the most inspiring passages I've ever read on the subject of vegetarianism: "We can't plead ignorance, only indifference. Those alive today are the generations that came to know better. We have the burden and the opportunity of living in the moment when the critique of factory farming broke into the popular consciousness. We are the ones of whom it will be fairly asked, What did you do when you learned the truth about eating animals?" In other words, we have all been handed the red pill. Will we swallow it?

The Happy Endings

I'm looking forward to a day when I have to shut our doors because there are no farm animals to rescue, when animal cruelty is an embarrassment of the past, when our society looks upon the mistreatment of animals the way it looks on the mistreatment of women or children or people with disabilities. And when no bubble is necessary. I have no illusions that I will see this change over-night. Cancer was a blip in my life compared with what I have ahead of me. It can feel overwhelming to work against such ingrained traditions and powerful interests, but I'm fighting for the day when people ultimately realize en masse that animals are here *with* us, not *for* us. Please join me in that fight.

We are the ones we've been waiting for.

—Hopi wisdom

Appendix:

An Opinionated
Lady's Opinions

Resources

Recommended Reading

Carol Adams's *The Sexual Politics of Meat* (Continuum, 1999).
A provocative and deep look at the connections among feminism, vegetarianism, animal defense, and literary theory. Her
Living Among Meat Eaters (Lantern, 2008) helps vegans get
perspective.

Jonathan Balcombe's *Pleasurable Kingdom* (Macmillan, 2007).
A pleasure to read! Full of research and anecdotes about animal behavior that we can only call pleasure.

Gene Baur's *Farm Sanctuary* (Simon & Schuster, 2007). The director of the first farmed-animal sanctuary in the United States
discusses his work and the lives of farm animals. It also tells the
story of factory farming, revealing its perverse logic and examining the havoc it wreaks.

T. Colin Campbell's *The China Study* (BenBella, 2006). Comparing
the dramatically different health issues between China and the

Appendix

United States over a twenty-year period, this book goes well beyond its medical findings into a realm that reveals the truth behind the special-interest groups, scientists, and government entities that have taken Americans down a deadly path.

Kris Carr's *Crazy Sexy Diet* (Skirt!, 2011). Fun, funny, and full of health info. Kris's path to overcoming cancer through a vegan diet and lifestyle change can be chronicled in her other books: *Crazy Sexy Cancer Survivor* and *Crazy Sexy Cancer Tips* (Skirt!, 2006, 2007).

Sue Coe's *Dead Meat* (Four Walls Eight Windows, 1995). A visual record of Coe's visits to forty slaughterhouses, cattle ranches, and hatcheries to document the grisly practices of the meat-packing industry.

Nick Cooney's *Change of Heart: What Psychology Can Teach Us About Spreading Social Change* (Lantern, 2010). A psychology primer for anyone wanting to make progressive change.

Karen Dawn's *Thanking the Monkey: Rethinking the Way We Treat Animals* (HarperCollins, 2008). Full of visual aids and cartoons; highly readable and comprehensive.

Gail Eisnitz's *Slaughterhouse: The Shocking Story of Greed, Neglect and Inhumane Treatment Inside the U.S. Meat Industry* (Prometheus, 2006). Gut-wrenching, yet carefully researched and documented.

Dr. Caldwell Esselstyn, Jr.'s *Prevent and Reverse Heart Disease* (Avery, 2007). Groundbreaking and assiduously researched; includes life-changing information and a lifesaving plan. The film and book *Forks over Knives* is based on the studies in this book.

Appendix

Jonathan Safran Foer's *Eating Animals* (Little, Brown, 2009). Beautifully written memoir-investigation by the acclaimed novelist. This exhaustively researched book, a tell-all of everything wrong with factory farms and commercial fishing, inspires and informs in a brilliant way.

Rory Freedman and Kim Barnouin's *Skinny Bitch* (Running Press, 2006) and their follow-up, one of the few vegan books directed specifically at men, *Skinny Bastard* (2009). Both are irreverent and hilarious—worth the hype.

Kathy Freston's *Veganist* (Weinstein, 2009). Helps readers think about "healthy living, conscious eating."

Colleen Patrick Goudreau's *The 30-Day Vegan Challenge: The Ultimate Guide to Eating Cleaner, Getting Leaner, and Living Compassionately* (Ballantine, 2011). The title says it all.

Amy Hatkoff's *The Inner World of Farm Animals* (Stewart, Tabori & Chang, 2009). Combines the latest research on the emotional and intellectual capacities of farm animals with touching stories to bring their inner world to life.

Melanie Joy's *Why We Love Dogs, Eat Pigs, and Wear Cows* (Canari, 2009). A groundbreaking book that explores the invisible system shaping our perception of the meat we eat, whereby we love some animals and eat others without knowing why.

Francis Moore Lappé's *Diet for a Small Planet* (Ballantine, 1991). One of the original powerful texts of the plant-based food movement, and it still holds up.

Howard Lyman's *Mad Cowboy: Plain Truth from the Cattle Rancher Who Won't Eat Meat* (Scribner, 2001). The erstwhile cattle rancher tells all.

Appendix

Erik Marcus's *Meat Market: Animals, Ethics, and Money* (Brio, 2005). Marcus presents a thorough examination of animal agriculture's cruelties and its far-reaching social costs. His *Vegan: The New Ethics of Eating* (McBooks, 2000) is a must-read guide for eating for your health, the environment, and the animals.

Jeffrey Moussaieff Masson's *The Face on Your Plate* and *The Pig Who Sang to the Moon* (Norton, 2010; Ballantine, 2004). The first shows how eating meat affects us ethically, environmentally, and health-wise; the second uncovers the emotional world of farm animals. Beautiful reads individually and together.

Laura Moretti's *All Heaven in a Rage* (MBK, 1999). This collection of essays, edited by Moretti, takes the blinders off regarding the unconscionable outrages of animal industry.

Ingrid Newkirk's *Making Kind Choices: Everyday Ways to Enhance Your Life Through Earth- and Animal Friendly Living* (St. Martin's, 2005). In this handbook, the founder and director of PETA shares easy ways to make choices that have a positive impact on the world.

No Voice Unheard's *Ninety-five: Meeting America's Farmed Animals in Stories and Photographs* (NVU, 2010). A collection of photographs and stories of rescued farm animals, including residents of WFAS.

Tom Regan's *The Case for Animal Rights* (University of California Press, 2004). A seminal text in the philosophy of the animal liberation movement.

John Robbins's *Diet for a New America*, *The Food Revolution*, and *The New Good Life* (H. J. Kramer, 1998; Conari, 2000; Ballantine, 2010). Classics of the veg writing genre, and for good—no, great—reason.

Appendix

Martin Rowe's *The Way of Compassion* (Lantern, 2000). These selections, edited by Rowe, link vegetarianism, animal rights, social justice, and environmentalism.

Matthew Scully's *Dominion* (St. Martin's, 2002). As smart and complete a treatment of the realities and philosophy of twenty-first-century agriculture as you'll read—and proves that veganism isn't just for lefties.

Alicia Silverstone's *The Kind Diet* (Rodale, 2009). Movie stars don't get more thoughtful and funny than this.

Peter Singer deserves a section of his own: I recommend his classic *Animal Liberation* and *In Defense of Animals: The Second Wave* (HarperCollins, 2009 [updated]; Blackwell, 2005), as well as the book he coauthored with Jim Mason, *The Ethics of What We Eat: Why Our Food Choices Matter* (Rodale, 2007).

Gene Stone's *Forks over Knives* (The Experiment, 2011). This is the companion book to the film of the same name—full of resources and recipes.

Will Tuttle's *The World Peace Diet* (Lantern, 2005). Takes veganism to a higher—by which I mean spiritual—level. A former Zen monk with a Ph.D. in education, Tuttle has worked extensively in intuition development, spiritual healing, meditation, music, creativity, vegan living, and cultural evolution.

Online Resources

Ellen DeGeneres's online guide to going vegan, Going Vegan with Ellen: vegan.ellen.warnerbros.com

Discerning Brute's fashion and food for "ethically handsome" men: discerningbrute.com

Appendix

Food and Water Watch, which works to ensure food safety: www
.foodandwaterwatch.org

Girly Girl Army's online everything eco, fashionable and vegan
guide: girliegirlarmy.com

Mercy for Animals' Choose Veg Guide: www.chooseveg.com

PETA's list of companies that do and don't test on animals:
www.peta.org/living/beauty-and-personal-care/companies/
default.aspx

Vegan Health's info on how to lead a healthy vegan lifestyle: www
.veganhealth.org

Vegetarian Resource Group's nutrition and health info: www.vrg.org

Woodstock Farm Animal Sanctuary website, of course! Information on how to adopt a vegan lifestyle, and on what's wrong with
animal agriculture; stories of our rescued animals; recipes;
information about visiting, sponsoring or adopting an animal,
staying at The Guesthouse at Woodstock Sanctuary, and much,
much more: woodstocksanctuary.org

Films

Bold Native (Denis Hennelly/Open Road Films, 2010). Indie feature
film whose main characters are animal rights activists on a
mission.

Earthlings (Shaun Monson/Nation Earth, 2005). A powerful and
informative documentary about society's treatment of animals,
narrated by Joaquin Phoenix with soundtrack by Moby.

Farm to Fridge (Lee Iorvino/Mercy for Animals, 2011; find it
online). As above, but with more recent investigative footage by
our friends at Mercy for Animals.

Appendix

Fast Food Nation: The Dark Side of the All-American Meal (Richard Linklater/Fox Searchlight, 2006). Based on the book by investigative journalist Eric Schlosser, examines the local and global influence of the U.S. fast-food industry.

Food, Inc. (Robert Kenner/Magnolia Pictures, 2008). This film lifts the veil on our nation's food industry, exposing the highly mechanized underbelly that has been hidden from the American consumer with the consent of our government's regulatory agencies, the USDA and FDA. In the end the film promotes "happy meat," which I'm clearly in disagreement with, but lots of good and well-presented information, regardless.

Forks over Knives (Lee Fulkerson/Monica Beach Media, 2011). Surgery's a lot more radical—and risky—and a lot less effective than adopting a healthy diet, as this powerful documentary makes clear.

Meet Your Meat (Bruce Friedrich/PETA, 2002; find it online). Seriously. If you're going to support the system, you should see what supporting it means.

Our Daily Bread (Nikolaus Geyrhalter/Icarus Films, 2005). A provocative documentary that offers an intensely clinical look at the machinery of industrial food production. Humans, animals, and crops appear incidentally, with droning conveyor belts, automated crop dusters, and other machinery in starring roles. This unusual film has no narration, dialogue, or music—just stoic tableaux that collectively tell a story.

Vegucated (Marisa Miller Wolfson/Filmbuff, 2011). This follows three meat-and-cheese-lovin' New Yorkers who agree to adopt a vegan diet for six weeks.

Appendix

My Favorite (Other!) Organizations

Animal Place: Farm animal sanctuary in Vacaville, California.

Animal Rescue and Protection League: Exposes animal cruelty and educates the public and policy makers to implement humane change.

ASPCA (American Society for the Prevention of Cruelty to Animals): The first humane organization in the Western Hemisphere.

Brighter Green: Policy "action tank" that raises awareness of environmental and animal issues.

Compassion over Killing: Animal advocacy organization working to end animal abuse.

Farm Sanctuary: The flagship farm animal sanctuary, located in Watkins Glen, New York, and Orland, California.

Food Empowerment Project: Educates about healthy food with a special focus on low-income communities and communities of color.

Humane League: Works to educate the public through public education, campaigns, and rescue.

Institute for Humane Education: Educational organization dedicated to creating a more humane world through training humane educators.

Jane Goodall Institute: Goodall's project empowers people around the globe to advocate for primates as well as humans and other animals.

Mercy for Animals: Dedicated to ending animal cruelty and to being a voice for animals through proactive consumer education and advertising campaigns, research and undercover investigations, rescues, working with news media, and grass-roots activism.

Our Hen House: Helps people find unique ways to change the world for animals.

Peaceful Prairie Sanctuary: Farm animal sanctuary in Deer Trail, Colorado.

Physicians Committee for Responsible Medicine: Group of health professionals that promotes a vegan diet and higher ethics and effectiveness in research, including an end to animal testing.

PETA (People for the Ethical Treatment of Animals): The largest animal rights organization in the world, focusing attention on animals used for food, entertainment, clothing, and experimentation.

Sea Shepherd: Works to end the destruction of habitat and slaughter of wildlife in the world's oceans, in order to conserve and protect ecosystems and species.

United Poultry Concerns: Rescue of and advocacy for domestic fowl; located in Machipongo, Virginia.

Vegan Outreach: Works to end animal exploitation through the promotion of a vegan lifestyle, especially through print materials.

VINE Sanctuary: Farmed and other animal sanctuary in Springfield, Vermont.

Other Sites to Check Out

ARconference.org: Annual animal rights conference registration and information.

Blossomnyc.com, Blossomdujour.com: Fabulous vegan eateries in New York City, from fast to fancy food.

Appendix

Cocoav.com: Gourmet handmade vegan chocolate shop in New York City.

Cosmosveganshoppe.com, Herbivore.com, Veganstore.com, The VegetarianSite.com, and VeganEssentials.com: Online shopping for ALL your vegan needs.

Jivamuktiyoga.com: My yoga practice, which incorporates animal rights.

Lanternbooks.com: Vegan books and more.

Lazydogcookies.com: Healthy, yummy vegan dog cookies.

MooShoes.com: Vegan shoe shop in New York City and online store.

Olsenhaus.com: Vegan shoe designer.

Stickyfingersbakery.com: Droolingly good vegan bakery in Washington, D.C., and online.

Vegantreats.com: Another drool-inducing vegan bakery in eastern Pennsylvania and online.

Vegnews.com: Vegan living magazine and website.

Worldpeaceinc.com: Info about their annual vegan yoga conference.

Restaurant Guides

HappyCow.net—a go-to source for veg and veg-friendly restaurants and stores worldwide. Includes maps, reviews, and links.

MoreThanSalad.com: Adds a Facebook-like element to adventures in vegan eating.

SuperVegan.com: Exhaustive guide to New York City (and area) veg and veg-friendly dining and food shopping.

VegDining.org: Same idea as Happy Cow; offers option to purchase a card that gives discounts at veg joints.

VegGuide.org: Same idea as Happy Cow.

Appendix

My Favorite Recipe Sources

COOKBOOKS

ALL of Isa Chandra Moskowitz and Terry Hope Romero's amazing collection of cookbooks: *Veganomicon: The Ultimate Vegan Cookbook*, *Vegan Cookies Invade Your Cookie Jar*, *Vegan Cupcakes Take Over the World*, and their newest, *Vegan Pie in the Sky*. Alone, Isa has also written *Vegan with a Vengeance*, *Vegan Brunch*, and *Appetite for Reduction*; and Terry has recently released the Latin-inspired *Viva Vegan!* (Da Capo).

The Artful Vegan by Eric Tucker with Bruce Enloe (Ten Speed, 2003). Want to wow the foodies in your life? This is the cookbook for you. Complex, nuanced, gourmet, and challenging.

The Candle Cafe Cookbook by Joy Pierson and Bart Potenza with Barbara Scott Goodman, and *The Candle 79 Cookbook* by Joy Pierson with Angel Ramos and Jorge Pineda (Clarkson Potter, 2003; Ten Speed, 2011). Bart and Joy are pioneers in award-winning veg dining—these books include many of their signature dishes.

The Conscious Cook by Tal Ronnen (William Morrow, 2009). A recent, impressive, and beautiful cookbook from the new hot vegan chef to the stars.

Don't Eat Me: A Cookbook for Animal Lovers by Robin Gager (Late Bloomers, 2010). Veganized versions of American classics, and color photos throughout of rescued animals at WFAS!

The Joy of Vegan Baking by Colleen Patrick-Goudreau (Four Winds, 2007). The definitive, must-have go-to cookbook for baking nerds.

Appendix

ONLINE RECIPES

Choosingraw.com: Tons of raw recipes, blog musings, and info on the raw diet.

Hellyeahitsvegan.com: Specializes in veganizing classic dishes.

Theppk.com: Isa Chandra Moskowitz's fun video and recipe treasure trove.

Vegalicious.com: The photos alone are worth a look, as are the high-class recipes.

Veganchef.com: Beverly Lynn Bennett's recipes and tips.

Veganlatina.com: Terry Hope Romero's blog and recipes.

Veganlunchbox.com: I wish my mom had had access to this website when I was a kid. . . .

Veganyumyum.com: Beautiful photos and recipes from Lauren Ulm.

VegWeb.com: Thousands of veg recipes, rated and heavily commented upon.

Some Tricks and Tips to Veganizing

I'm a good cook, though I rarely have time anymore. I like to cook, and I love having large dinner parties, something I share with my husband (although he doesn't like the cleaning part so much). Here are some of the veggie weapons in my plant-based arsenal; most are available in health food stores or well-stocked supermarkets:

Vegenaise. This is a replacement for regular mayonnaise and is so good, a lot of my non-veg friends still prefer it over the "real" stuff. I use it in mock chicken salad, on sandwiches, and in salad dressings and aioli.

Nutritional yeast. We buy it from the bulk section in our co-op, and I sprinkle it on pasta or popcorn for a cheesy experience. You can combine it with the nondairy milk of your choice and a little flour, and it forms the basis of any kind of cream sauce. Nutritional yeast is very high in vitamin B complex. Our dogs love it, too.

Extra-firm tofu. This is not your mother's mushy, gelatinous tofu. It now comes in many different textures, and you can even cheat and buy pre-marinated. See the recipes section for a basic tofu scramble dish that is an easy crowd-pleaser.

Daiya. This preshredded "cheese" is a very close analog to the kind of cheese you'd have in a burrito or on pizza. It's unusual in that it's based on tapioca, not soy. A common mistake is to use too much. Since Daiya's flavor is rather intense, I advise adding about half of the amount you'd normally use with real cheese, which is also good for your muffin top (if you have one).

Truffle oil. The tiniest drizzle of this tasty stuff on pasta or a pizza just before serving will take it to a new level. Don't worry; although some dogs are used to find truffle mushrooms, the truffle oils you and I can afford are generally flavored synthetically.

Whipped garlic. OMG if you like garlic and are lucky enough to have a Lebanese or Mediterranean take-out place near you, stock your freezer with this stuff. When a dollop of this is added to a sandwich or almost any dish, the meal gains a garlicky goodness that warms my heart (and challenges my lower intestine, but *so* worth it!). I've never been able to make it successfully at home, but Google tells me that the secret is to add lemon at the end.

Kale. Kale is so freakin' good for you. Lots of people love it, but lots of people don't. Try tossing it with your favorite dressing, perhaps something with a little sweetness to offset kale's bitterness. If you massage it with your hands, it becomes a new thing—the dreaded toughness disappears and it's great. For a quick and tasty kale salad, add some or all of the following: minced red onion; any kind of nut (walnuts or cashews are good choices); shredded carrot; and dried fruit, like currants or cranberries.

Avocados. I adore them *so* much. I love to make a salad dressing out of them, just blending one up with a good squeeze of lemon, a dash of salt, and a glug of olive oil (good on kale).

Frozen fruit. A common breakfast for a busy gal on the go is a quick smoothie, and frozen fruit is an absolute staple to have on hand. You can use OJ or almond milk as a base. Toss the frozen fruit and the OJ or nondairy milk in a blender and blend the snot out of it. For the fruit, you can sub a fresh or frozen banana. Try to buy organic fruit if it's available.

Raw cashews. Can be soaked and blended to make a really amazing cheese substitute. Add red pepper, lemon juice, onion powder, and sea salt, and voilà! A healthy (it's the good fat) vegan cheese. If you add water to them in the blender, you get a delicious cream. Recipes can be found easily online.

Quinoa. This grain is hard to spell and say (KEEN-wha), but it has almost every vowel you need to get you through the day. It tastes like a cousin of couscous; it is super high in nutrients and cooks fast. Use it in place of rice. Or let this magical grain cool and add it to salad. For extra flavor add some . . .

Better Than Bouillon. Sold in a little jar, this veggie bouillon packs a lot of flavor. Add a heaping teaspoon to the water when making your quinoa and it'll knock your Birkenstocks off, you hippie. You can also get premade veggie stock, but BTB has a nice intensity that I really like.

Lizano Salsa sauce. This particular Costa Rican condiment is tough to find in the United States, although in Costa Rica it's as common as ketchup. We order it online. It'll add zing to any kind of bean-based or Mexican dish you're making. It's a must on our tofu scramble, as is . . .

Turmeric. The essential ingredient in a tofu scramble, this spice transforms the tofu to an enticing shade of yellow and adds a nice, unique flavor. Season to taste.

My Favorite Animal-Product Substitutes
There's a dizzying amount of delectable substitutes these days, and the list grows longer all the time. All those options can be overwhelming, so while I recommend that you try anything and

everything you can, you may want to start with these excellent products:

Butter. Earth Balance.

Mayonnaise. As mentioned above, the best is Vegenaise.

Ice cream. Organic Nectars, Coconut Bliss, So Delicious.

Cheese. Daiya, Dr-Cow.

Coffee creamer. Wildwood.

Soy milk. Silk.

Almond milk. Almond Breeze.

Coconut milk. So Delicious.

Eggnog. Silk Nog.

Cold cuts. Field Roast, Tofurky.

Faux ground beef and chicken. Savage River Farms products, Boca Ground Crumbles, Match Meats.

Sausage. Field Roast, Tofurky.

Egg replacer. Ener-G.

Recipes

Except for the very last, these recipes are compliments of cowriter Gretchen Primack, a fabulous cook, who makes me very happy when she feeds me. Here are some of her favorites, in her words.

Cheesy Lasagna

My favorite lasagna, for which I get frequent requests. It's extremely challenging to stop eating this. Modified from a recipe I found on vegweb.com.

Makes one 11 x 7-inch lasagna

½ pound cauliflower or other veggies (optional)

1 tablespoon olive oil

6 cloves garlic, peeled and minced (I love garlic! Adjust the amount down if you don't.)

½ pound mushrooms, sliced

2 teaspoons Italian herb blend

1 pound extra-firm tofu

1 8-ounce container Tofutti vegan cream cheese

2 tablespoons lemon juice

⅛ teaspoon nutmeg

⅓ cup nutritional yeast

Salt and pepper, to taste

1 or 2 jars of your favorite spaghetti sauce

15 lasagna noodles, prepared according to instructions

5-ounce bag fresh spinach leaves (I like to use baby spinach.)

Bread crumbs, fresh basil, or vegan parmesan (optional)

Preheat the oven to 375 degrees.

Slice the cauliflower or other veggie and steam for a few minutes until soft and then set aside.

Put the olive oil in a large skillet; place over a medium-high heat. When the oil is hot, add the garlic and mushrooms and sauté for about 3 minutes, or until the garlic is slightly browned. Add the herbs, tofu, vegan cream cheese, and lemon juice; stir constantly until the cream cheese melts. Remove the skillet from the heat and stir in the nutmeg and nutritional yeast. Add salt and pepper, to taste.

Spread enough spaghetti sauce to coat the bottom of an 11 x 7-inch baking dish. Add three noodles. Spread the cream cheese mixture over the noodles. Place three noodles on top of that and spread more spaghetti sauce, then add a generous layer of spinach (it cooks down more than you think). Repeat until all the noodles are used up, then top with spaghetti sauce. Feel free to sprinkle the top with bread crumbs, herbs, and/or vegan parmesan.

Cover the baking dish (easiest with a cookie sheet) and bake for 15 minutes. Uncover and bake for an additional 20 to 30 minutes, or until the lasagna is heated all the way through. DELICIOUS!

Insanely Tasty *VegNews* Mac 'n' Cheese

VegNews magazine is a recipe (and article) powerhouse, and
this recipe was originally published in its pages. There are a lot
of great vegan mac 'n' cheese recipes out there, so I recommend
you try a few, but this is my favorite. I tend to double the garlic
and Dijon mustard, and I always add about ⅓ cup nutritional
yeast for extra "cheesiness," B vitamins, minerals, and protein.

Serves 4 to 6

4 quarts water

1 tablespoon sea salt

8 ounces macaroni

4 slices of bread, torn into
 large pieces

2 tablespoons plus ⅓ cup
 Earth Balance butter
 substitute, divided

2 tablespoons chopped
 shallot

1 cup chopped red or yellow
 potato

¼ cup chopped carrot

⅓ cup chopped onion

1 cup water

¼ cup raw cashews

2 teaspoons sea salt

½ teaspoon minced garlic

1 teaspoon Dijon mustard

1 tablespoon freshly
 squeezed lemon juice

¼ teaspoon black pepper

⅛ teaspoon cayenne

⅓ cup nutritional yeast
 (optional)

¼ teaspoon paprika

Preheat the oven to 350 degrees.

In a large pot, bring the 4 quarts water and 1 tablespoon salt to a boil. Add the macaroni and cook until just al dente. Drain the pasta and rinse with cold water. Set aside.

In a food processor, make bread crumbs by pulverizing the bread and 2 tablespoons of the butter substitute to a medium-fine texture. Set aside.

In a saucepan, place shallot, potato, carrot, onion, and 1 cup water, and bring to a boil. Cover the pan and simmer for 15 minutes, or until vegetables are very soft.

In a blender, process the cashews, 2 teaspoons salt, garlic, remainder of the butter substitute, mustard, lemon juice, black pepper, and cayenne. Add the softened vegetables and their cooking water to the blender (along with the nutritional yeast, if you want) and process until perfectly smooth.

In a large bowl, toss the cooked pasta and blended cheese sauce until completely coated. Spread mixture into a casserole dish, sprinkle with prepared bread crumbs, and dust with paprika. Bake for 30 minutes or until the cheese sauce is bubbling and the top has turned golden brown.

Quick Savory Nut Loaf

Want to make your dinner guests swoon on an autumn or winter night? Serve this recipe, adapted from Rose Elliot's The Complete Vegetarian Cuisine, *with roasted potatoes. FLAT-OUT SWOON. I've watched people fight over the last slice.*

Serves 4 to 6 (double or triple it for a crowd)

4 tablespoons Earth Balance butter substitute (or other brand, but this is by far my favorite)

2 large onions, peeled and finely chopped

1 teaspoon dried thyme

1 tablespoon whole wheat flour

½ cup water

1 cup cashews, finely ground

1 cup hazelnuts, walnuts, or other nut of your choice, finely ground

1⅓ cup whole wheat bread crumbs

Ener-G egg replacer equivalent of 2 eggs (optional)

1 tablespoon lemon juice

Salt and pepper, to taste

Preheat the oven to 400 degrees.

Melt the butter substitute in a large saucepan, add onions, and sauté gently for 10 minutes or until the onions are very tender.

Add the thyme and flour, stir for 2 minutes, then add the water and stir until thickened.

Remove from heat, add cashews and hazelnuts, bread crumbs, egg replacer, lemon juice, and salt and pepper, to taste. Mix well.

Pack the nut loaf mixture in a well-oiled pan and baste with oil of your choosing (such as canola, grape-seed, or surf lower).

Bake for 45 minutes to an hour, depending how dark and rich you want the loaf.

Bonus: My Delicious, Easy Gravy

Makes 2 cups

2 tablespoons Earth Balance butter substitute	**½ cup chopped mushrooms**
1 small yellow onion, finely chopped	**2 tablespoons flour**
	2 cups vegetable stock
	Spices, to taste

Melt a tablespoon or two of Earth Balance butter substitute in a skillet over medium heat and add a finely chopped onion. Sauté until the onion is soft and translucent, about 8 minutes. Add a handful of chopped mushrooms—try cremini for a fancy turn, but white button work fine—and sauté an extra three minutes. Add 2 tablespoons flour, and sauté until the flour browns. Add a few pinches of sage or thyme at this stage. Then add 2 cups veggie stock, raise the heat to bring to a boil, turn the heat back down, and stir gently on medium-low until the mixture thickens. Lovely.

Almond Feta Cheese with Herb Oil

Rich, decadent, scrumptious cheese from Vegetarian Times *magazine, which says, "Unbaked, it will be smooth and spreadable. Baking will make it a bit more crumbly, like traditional feta." I'm just as likely to not bake it, forgo the herbs, and serve it with crackers, but both ways are marvelous.*

Makes one 10-ounce round

1 cup whole blanched almonds, soaked overnight in cold water	1¼ teaspoon salt
	½ cup cold water
¼ cup lemon juice	1 tablespoon fresh thyme leaves
3 tablespoon plus ¼ cup olive oil, divided	1 teaspoon fresh rosemary leaves
1 clove garlic, peeled	

Drain the soaking liquid from the almonds, rinse them under cold running water, and drain again.

In a food processor, purée the almonds, lemon juice, 3 tablespoons oil, garlic, salt, and cold water for 6 minutes, or until very smooth and creamy.

Place a large strainer over a bowl, and line with a triple layer of cheesecloth. Spoon the almond mixture into the cheesecloth. Bring the corners and sides of the cloth together, and twist around the mixture, forming into an orange-size ball and squeezing to help extract moisture. Secure with a rubber band or kitchen twine. Chill in the refrigerator for 12 hours, or overnight. Discard excess liquid.

After the ball has chilled, preheat the oven to 200 degrees. Line a baking sheet with parchment paper. Unwrap cheese (it will be soft), and transfer it from the cheesecloth to the prepared baking sheet. Flatten the ball to form a 6-inch round, about ¾ inch thick. Bake for 40 minutes, or until the top is slightly firm. Cool, then chill. (Cheese can be made up to this point two days ahead; keep refrigerated.)

Combine the remaining cup oil, thyme, and rosemary in a small saucepan. Warm oil over a medium-low heat for 2 minutes, or until the oil is very hot but not simmering. Cool to room temperature. Drizzle the herb oil over the cheese just before serving.

Cashew Pumpkin Tartlets

We are SO LUCKY to have a fantastic vegan restaurant right in Woodstock, the Garden Cafe on the Green. I don't know what we'd do without it or chef Pam Brown's wonderful recipes. This one is deceptively simple to make but worthy of a special occasion.

Makes 4 to 6 tartlets, depending on size (mini tart pans or ramekins)

2 cups raw cashews, plus extra for garnish

1 8-ounce container vegan cream cheese

1 15-ounce can plain pumpkin purée

1 tablespoon fresh sage, or 1 teaspoon dried

2 teaspoon miso (barley or mellow)

1 teaspoon canola oil

Preheat the oven to 350 degrees.

In a food processor, grind the 2 cups cashews until they become a powder. Add the rest of the ingredients and blend again until creamy, scraping down the sides of the processor to mix well. Spray tart pans or ramekins cups and fill. Smooth the tops with a knife to even. Press a few cashews into each tart.

Bake for 25 minutes or until the tarts are brown on top.

Speedy yet Heavenly Thai Basil Sesame Noodles

This is an Asian twist on pesto. Very intense, just how I like things. I found it on PETA's website, a great recipe source.

Serves 4

1 12-ounce package rice noodles

1 cup fresh basil leaves

2 tablespoons sesame seeds (black if you can find them), plus more for garnish

5 garlic cloves, peeled

1 teaspoon sesame oil

1 tablespoon soy sauce

1 tablespoon fresh lime juice

½ tablespoon red pepper flakes

¼ cup olive oil

Salt, to taste

Cook the noodles according to the package directions. Drain.

In a food processor, combine the basil, sesame seeds, garlic, sesame oil, soy sauce, lime juice, and red pepper. With the processor running, gradually add the olive oil until mixture is combined and slightly thickened. Season with the salt.

Toss the noodles with the sauce. Garnish with sesame seeds—the black ones are especially dramatic here.

Best Chocolate Cake Ever

This recipe has been floating around forever, so I'm not sure whom to attribute it to. All I know is that you can throw away every other chocolate cake recipe you have, forever. And it takes only five minutes, plus the baking time! Joyously enough, this recipe also easily doubles to make a classic layer cake.

Makes one moist, delicious 9-inch cake

1½ cups flour	1 teaspoon vanilla extract
1 cup sugar	1 tablespoon white vinegar
1 teaspoon baking soda	5 tablespoons vegetable oil
1 teaspoon salt	1 cup water
4 tablespoons cocoa powder	

Preheat the oven to 350 degrees.

In a large mixing bowl, sift or whisk the dry ingredients together into a mound.

Make three wells in the mound, put the vanilla in one, vinegar in another, and oil in the third. Slowly pour in the water, mixing only as much as necessary to get most of the lumps out of the batter.

Transfer the batter to a greased and floured 9-inch cake pan and bake for 25 minutes. The cake is done when a knife comes out of the center clean. Let cool completely before frosting.

Simple yet Lovely Fudgy Frosting

Care of my friend Kirsti Gholson—a breeze to whip up, but worthy of the divine cake underneath.

Makes enough to frost one double-layer cake

- ½ cup Earth Balance butter substitute (Once you try it, you'll say good-bye to butter!)
- ⅓ cup plain or vanilla soy milk
- 1 teaspoon vanilla
- ⅔ cup cocoa powder
- 3 cups powdered sugar
- 1 tablespoon liqueur (optional)

Heat the butter substitute in a microwave or on a stovetop until just melted, and then add the soy milk, vanilla, and liqueur (if using). Whisk in the cocoa and sugar. Add more sugar or soy milk if necessary, until the frosting reaches a creamy, velvety consistency.

Blueberry-Lemon Corn Biscuit Cobbler

Isa Chandra Moskowitz and Terry Hope Romero have produced a number of absolutely essential cooking and baking books, most recently Vegan Pie in the Sky. *This is one of my favorite recipes from it—ambrosial, original, crowd-pleasing, and not hard to make, either.*

Serves 6 to 8

5 cups frozen blueberries, unthawed

2 tablespoons fresh lemon juice

⅓ cup sugar

4 teaspoons tapioca powder or cornstarch

½ teaspoon ground cinnamon

¾ cup unbleached flour

½ cup yellow cornmeal

¼ cup sugar

1½ teaspoons baking powder

¼ teaspoon baking soda

Pinch of salt

4 tablespoons cold nonhydrogenated margarine

2 tablespoons soy milk

2 tablespoons lemon juice

Grated zest of 1 lemon

1 teaspoon sugar

Preheat the oven to 400 degrees.

In a 10-inch deep-dish ceramic pie plate combine the frozen berries, lemon juice, ⅓ cup sugar, tapioca powder or cornstarch, and cinnamon. Transfer to the oven and bake for 25 minutes, then remove from the oven. Leave the oven on; you'll need it again.

Ten minutes before removing the berry mixture from the oven, make the biscuit topping: In a large mixing bowl, stir together the flour, cornmeal, ¼ cup sugar, baking powder, baking soda, and salt. Using a pastry cutter or your fingers, cut the margarine into the flour mixture until the mixture looks crumbly. In a measuring cup, stir together the soy milk, lemon juice, and lemon zest, then sprinkle it over the dry ingredients and stir just enough to moisten ingredients to form a soft dough.

Gently gather the dough into a ball and, on a lightly floured surface, pat it into a rectangle about 1 inch thick.

Use a sharp knife to slice the rectangle into eight equal squares, then arrange the dough squares on top of the hot blueberry mixture, spacing them evenly. Sprinkle the cobbler with 1 teaspoon sugar.

Bake for another 20 to 22 minutes, until the biscuits are lightly browned and firm. Remove the cobbler from the oven, let it cool for 10 minutes, then serve warm with vegan whipped topping or vegan vanilla ice cream.

Coffee Chocolate Tart

I found this on the VegNews *website, and it is heaven. It was originally assembled by Becky Stern of* Craft *magazine, and she therefore rocks my world. Suitable for special occasions, to be sure.*

Serves 12

For the crust:
½ **cup butter substitute**
    (such as Earth Balance)
⅓ **cup sugar**
1 **teaspoon vanilla**
¾ **cup walnuts, finely**
    chopped
1½ **cups all-purpose flour**

For the filling:
1 **cup chopped bittersweet**
    chocolate
1¼ **cups coffee**
1 **tablespoon cornstarch**
1 **teaspoon vanilla**
¼ **teaspoon salt**
⅓ **cup slivered almonds**
    (optional)

Preheat the oven to 350 degrees.

In a medium bowl, cream the butter substitute and sugar until light and fluffy. Add the vanilla and walnuts and blend. Mix in flour ⅓ cup at a time until dough sticks together and is slightly moist.

Press the dough with your fingertips into an ungreased tart pan. Bake until the edges are just barely starting to brown, about 20 minutes. Allow crust to cool completely before filling.

For the filling, in a small pot, melt chocolate on low heat on the stove or in the microwave until it softens. In another small pot, bring coffee to a gentle boil. Pour over the softened chocolate and stir the mixture until smooth. Add the cornstarch, vanilla, and salt.

Pour the filling into the cooled crust. Place the tart in the refrigerator and chill for six hours. Decorate the top with slivered almonds—running them along the edge of the crust, for instance, looks snazzy. To serve, I recommend dipping a sharp knife in hot water before you slice each wedge.

Jenny's Husband Doug's Easy, Free-Form Tofu Scramble

Husbands and boyfriends everywhere will make their significant others very happy when this is served in bed.

Serves 4

1 package firm, extra-firm, or super-firm tofu, drained

1 tablespoon light oil

1 medium onion, chopped

1 bell pepper of any color, chopped (optional)

2 carrots, chopped (optional)

3 cloves of garlic, peeled and crushed

Variety of vegetables of your choice (optional; see instructions below)

Lizano Salsa sauce (see p. 243) or condiment of choice

Any of your favorite spices

1 teaspoon turmeric

Nutritional yeast, or nondairy cheese of your choice

Salt and pepper, to taste

Hot sauce, to taste

Slice the tofu into approximately ¾-inch slabs, arrange in a row, wrap in paper towels and then kitchen towels, and place under a heavy object like a cast-iron skillet or a phone book (remember those?) to squeeze out any excess water.

In oil, brown the onion, and pepper and carrots if desired, or cara-melize them for extra flavor. Hand-crumble the tofu into the pan and add garlic, and stir for a few minutes so it begins to brown. Use a tiny bit of water and a spatula to loosen and scrape up the yummy browned bits and prevent sticking. Add any or all of the following: frozen green peas or corn, thawed under hot water tap; kale, spin-ach, or any other cooking green, chopped; zucchini or yellow squash; or pretty much any vegetable you can imagine, factoring in cooking time. Use common sense here—squishy veggies like toma-toes should be added toward the end, tougher ones like broccoli toward the beginning. (You can also add things like veggie sau-sages or even diced, fried potatoes to bulk it up for a larger crowd.)

As everything cooks over medium heat, start to add some sauce for flavor. Lizano is great because it's not too spicy. If you don't have that, use veggie Worcestershire sauce or (lightly) soy sauce. Add any spices you want—oregano and red pepper flakes are my usual favorites.

Last, add a teaspoon or so of turmeric, which adds a cool yellow color, and for the important cheesy flavor sprinkle in a few table-spoons of nutritional yeast or a nondairy cheese such as Daiya. Season with salt and pepper and hot sauce as you like, and load up in a tortilla wrap, or over toast, or just in a bowl!

Acknowledgments

....

First and foremost, always I want to acknowledge my husband, whose love, support, tireless energy, humor, friendship, and shared passion have made Woodstock Farm Animal Sanctuary possible. As with a tandem bike, I could never do this work without him pedaling along with me. I want to thank and acknowledge my wonderful and supportive mother, Judy, and sister, Loren, whom I love dearly and am thankful to have as my core family, along with my loving grandparents, Tom and Patsy Pittman, and forever cool uncle, Mike Pittman. I am grateful as well to my mother-in-law, Carole Abel, who lent her wisdom and guidance as a retired literary agent.

I am grateful as well to my cowriter and friend Gretchen Primack, who nailed the structure so well in the proposal that we never looked back—and whose patience, passion, nagging, and knowledge were what I needed to get this book done; to Linda Loewenthal, my wonderful agent at the David Black Agency in New York City; and to my editor, Megan Newman, my publicist, Beth

Acknowledgments

Parker, and to Miriam Rich, Andrea Ho, Gigi Campo, and the rest of the wonderful team at Avery Boooks.

We've had a small but very busy Board of Directors helping the sanctuary grow as fast as it has. Close friends Dawn Ladd and Eva Orlowski in particular have gone beyond all expectations and have braved late nights and stained car interiors in our efforts to help animals. Dawn served with her unique blend of Swiss-Army-knife-like talents for over half a decade and Eva still provides an organizational force that keeps us on track. More recently J. L. Fields and Cynthia King have joined us and have already proven their great commitment to both WFAS and farmed animals.

To Susie Coston, the shelter director at Farm Sanctuary and the person who, famously, picked up a pig turd with her bare hands, I owe all my initial knowledge of farm animal care. She is a dear friend and true hero to farm animals and to many of us who know her.

At the time of writing, we now have an incredible all-vegan staff of nine (including Doug and me). On the farm are Farm Manager Sheila Hyslop, Animal Caregivers Dawnell Kilbourne, Jodie Sidote, and Hervé Breuil, and Maintenance Manager Dave Miller. On the administrative side we have Natalie Alcalde keeping our finances in order and Elana Kirshenbaum coordinating our programs, volunteers, and animal placement. I'm so thankful that I work with a group of people who care about animals and the mission of WFAS as much as I do. They are all comrades in the movement.

We have also been fortunate to have had *seriously incredible* volunteers and friends who have been like unpaid staff in the past and present: Sheila Hyslop (before joining our staff just last year), Mike and Wendy Stura, Chris Kerr, Mike Radzvilowicz, Lourdes

Acknowledgments

Jovel, Jean Rhode, Stevie Jones, Bob Esposito—these are the folks who have dedicated huge amounts of time and energy and have shaped who we are today.

Then we have our past staff who have cared for and loved the animals and worked their butts off in doing so, and then moved on to *vastly inferior jobs* (I'm kidding): Robin Henderson Williams, Amber Plaut, Phil Deyman, Rebecca Moore, Rachel Winograd, Anthony DeSimone, and Sophie Keel. They will always be a part of the WFAS extended family.

Many other volunteers come as often as they can to lend a hand, or make a special trip to stay in the area and volunteer for us for days at a time. To all of them we are so very thankful!

Space doesn't permit individual descriptions, but I am eternally grateful to these friends, volunteers, and supporters who have done wonderful, generous things for Woodstock Farm Animal Sanctuary: Anthony Acock, Ahimsa Foundation, Nancy Andreassi, Abbe Aronson, Joy Askew, the ASPCA, the George F. Baker Trust, Gene Baur, Pamela Blackwell, Tracy Bonham, Jeffrey Braverman, Pam Brown, Kris Carr, the Michele and Agnes Cestone Foundation, Cat Clyne, Jonathan Donahue, Len Egert, Dawn Ellsworth, the Blanche Enders Charitable Trust, Michael Festa, Jason Fine, Robin Flynn, the Nalith Foundation, Kelly Galligan, Sharon Gannon and David Life, Kirsti Gholson, Brad Goldberg, George and Nancy Goldner, Derek Goodwin, the Max and Lili Hahn Memorial Fund, Susan Hammersley, Scott and Gina Hertzog, Nemo Hoffman, the Lauren Horowitz Charitable Fund, Chrissie Hynde, Janice Ianelli, Jim James, Cassie Karopkin, David Karopkin, Petrina Katsikas, Julie Kirkpatrick, Danielle Konya, Erica and Sara Kubersky, Sean Lennon, Jeff Mangum, Libra Max, Jenna McDavid, Nellie McKay, Jason

Acknowledgments

and Cayce Mell, Heidi Miller, Heather Mills, Rohit Misra, Elizabeth Mitchell, Moby, Gali Neufeld, the Om Foundation, the William and Charlotte Parks Foundation, Joanne Pearson, Nancy Pearson, Elvis Perkins, Dan Piraro, Cheryl Radzvilowicz, Martin Rowe, Kathy Ruttenberg, Amy Sacks, Fernanda Santos, Adam Sender, Brian Shapiro, Paul Shapiro, Roni Shapiro, the Shutz Engel Trust, David and Sheri Silver, Ashley Lou Smith, Andrea Barrist Stern, Anne Sullivan, Astra Taylor, Anne Marie Tortorelli, Joey Trachtman, Amy Trakinski, Sue Troutman, *VegNews*, the Winley Foundation, Brett and Jaime Wyker, Lauri Ylvisaker, and WAMC, WDST, and WKZE.

Finally, I'd like to thank Cam MacQueen, the employee of PETA whom I met at the Chicago Diner in 1993 and who gave me the chance to get involved and *do something*. And to my cat Boogie (1980–1998), who opened my eyes to the souls within our fellow animals.

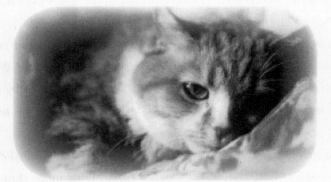

Be A Part of It—Join Us!

....

Woodstock Farm Animal Sanctuary (WFAS) is a 501(c)(3) charitable organization and shelter that works to end the systematic abuse of animals used for food. At the heart of our mission is the hands-on work of rescuing, rehabilitating, and caring for farm animal refugees—as well as educating the public about the treatment of animals who are raised for food and the many benefits of a plant-based diet.

If you have been moved by hearing my story or by what you've learned about the plight of farmed animals or the work of WFAS, you can support our work by making a donation online or by mail, becoming a member, sponsoring an animal, or simply by telling others about WFAS.

The majority of our support comes from individuals *like you* who believe in our work and our message. With more than two hundred animals in our care, we need your support for them, for the ones still to be rescued, and for the billions of farmed animals everywhere for whom we strive to be a voice.

Be A Part of It—Join Us!

Please visit WFAS in Woodstock, New York, during our hours of operation: Saturdays and Sundays from 11:00 a.m. to 4:00 p.m., April through October.

Woodstock Farm Animal Sanctuary

P.O. Box 1329

Woodstock, NY 12498

845-679-5955

www.woodstocksanctuary.org

Notes

....

2. The Flying Leg

Page 26 Shipping regulations say nothing about food, water, weather: United States Postal Service regulations 326.3 and 326.4.

Page 32 I had no idea that McDonald's is the world's largest purchaser of beef": Eric Schlosser, *Fast Food Nation: The Dark Side of the All-American Meal* (New York: Houghton Mifflin, 2001), 204.

Page 32 I didn't know that many of those are dairy cows: Ibid.

Page 32 I had no idea that for its McChicken sandwich: Karen Dawn, *Thanking the Monkey* (New York: HarperCollins, 2008), 130.

Page 33 I had no idea that McDonald's suppliers: Danielle Nierenberg, *Happier Meals: Rethinking the Global Meat Industry* (Washington, DC: Worldwatch Institute, 2005), 58–59.

3. Taking the Red Pill

Page 38 A lot of the discussions about animal welfare and rights: Tony Weis, "Breadbasket Contradictions," in Geoffrey Lawrence, Kristen Lyons, and Tabatha Wallington, eds., *Food Security, Nutrition, and Sustainability* (London: Earthscan, 2010), 29.

Notes

Page 41 "There's a schizoid quality to our relationship": Michael Pollan, *The Omnivore's Dilemma* (New York: Penguin, 2006), 306.

Page 42 These are just some examples: Jonathan Safran Foer, *Eating Animals* (New York: Little, Brown, 2009), 64–65. "The Hidden Lives of Pigs," People for the Ethical Treatment of Animals website. http://www.peta.org/issues/animals-used-for-food/hidden-lives-pigs.aspx. Accessed June 18, 2011.

Page 43 "The question is not, can they reason?": Jeremy Bentham, *An Introduction to the Principles of Morals and Legislation* (Oxford: Clarendon Press, 1879), 311.

Page 45 The researchers could determine lethal doses: Dawn, *Thanking the Monkey*, 216–17.

Page 45 Animal studies for cancer are notoriously unreliable: Dr. Neal Barnard, "A Look at Cancer Research," Physicians Committee for Responsible Medicine, http://www.pcrm.org/resch/humres/cancer research.html. Accessed June 7, 2011.

Page 45 Animal bodies are different enough from ours: C. Ray Greek and Jean Greek, *Specious Science: How Genetics and Evolution Reveal Why Medical Research on Animals Harms Humans* (New York: Continuum, 2002), 106–25.

Page 45 "What, pray tell, makes us think that a mouse is . . . ?": Quoted in Dawn, *Thanking the Monkey*, 218–19.

Page 46 Plenty of drugs that passed muster: See C. Ray Greek and Jean Greek, *Sacred Cows and Golden Geese* (New York: Continuum, 2001), and their *Specious Science*.

Page 47 Mercifully, some companies don't test at all: "Position Paper on Animal Research," Physicians Committee for Responsible Medicine website, July 2010. http://www.pcrm.org/resch/anexp/index.html. Accessed March 23, 2011.

Page 47 L'Oréal now tests skin care products: "R&D Collaboration Aims to Develop Alternative to Animal Testing," Cosmetics Design Europe website, January 2010. http://www.cosmeticsdesign-europe.com/For

Notes

mulation-Science/R-D-collaboration-aims-to-develop-alternative-to-animal-testing. Accessed May 14, 2011.

Page 47 And yet major companies like Colgate-Palmolive: Dawn, *Thanking the Monkey*, 240–41.

Page 48 I read about tests in which animals are strapped down: Ibid.

Page 48 "'oral gavage'": "What Do They Test?" Stop Huntington Life Sciences website. http://www.shac.net/HLS/what_tests.html. Accessed May 19, 2011.

Page 48 I'd also read about chemicals injected: R. D. Ryder, *Victims of Science: The Use of Animals in Research* (Don Mills, Ontario: Burns & MacEachern, 1975).

Page 49 I read about their complex matriarch-led families: G. A. Bradshaw, *Elephants on the Edge: What Animals Teach Us About Humanity* (New Haven, CT: Yale University Press, 2009).

Page 50 As a result, of course, these animals are deeply distressed: "Mercy for Animals Spotlights Circus Cruelty," Mercy for Animals website.http://www.mercyforanimals.org/5outrage03.html. Accessed July 3, 2011.

Page 50 As soon as I'd written and delivered that speech, I had to turn my research attention: Dawn, *Thanking the Monkey*, 129–30.

Page 51 This would be bad enough: "Animal Behaviour: Chickens Feel for Each Other," *Nature* 471 (March 2011), 268.

Page 52 HRW published an exhaustive study: Lance A. Compa, "Blood, Sweat, and Fear: Workers' Rights in U.S. Meat and Poultry Plants," Human Rights Watch, Articles and Chapters, Paper 331, 2004. http://digitalcommons.ilr.cornell.edu/articles/331/.

Page 54 They have nerve endings and feel pain: Foer, *Eating Animals*, 65.

Page 54 Killing them unnecessarily for food: Ibid., 189.

Page 55 "Now at last I can look at you in peace": Max Brod, *Franz Kafka: A Biography* (New York: Da Capo, 1995), 84.

Notes

4. The Horrible Bunny

Page 59 "We must fight against the spirit of unconscious cruelty: Venkata Ramana, ed., *The Book of Uncommon Quips and Quotations* (New Delhi: Pustak Mahal, 2005), 100.

Page 60 Unbeknownst to most of its residents, New York City: Anne Barnard, "Meeting, then Eating, the Goat," *New York Times*, May 24, 2009.

Page 60 These small, local markets are in some ways the opposite: "PETA Reveals Extreme Cruelty at Kosher Slaughterhouses," People for the Ethical Treatment of Animals website. http://www.peta.org/features/agriprocessors.aspx. Accessed August 27, 2011.

Page 60 So, along with raising serious ethical questions: D. A. Senne et al., "Live Poultry Markets: The Missing Link in the Epidemiology of Avian Influenza," *Proceedings of the Third International Symposium on Avian Influenza* (Richmond, VA: U.S. Animal Health Association, 1992).

Page 67 On the other end were Doug and his mom: Fernanda Santos, "A Rescued Goat Gets a Chance for a Normal Life," *New York Times*, May 1, 2008.

Page 69 But this story was something different: Mark Scarbrough and Bruce Weinstein, "Goat: The Final Frontier," *Washington Post*, April 5, 2011. http://www.washingtonpost.com/lifestyle/food/goat-meat-the-final-frontier/2011/03/28/AF0p2OjC_story.html.

Page 75 "a failure, in attitude or practice": Joan Dunayer, *Speciesism* (New York: Lantern, 2004).

Page 84 Pregnant horses, scientists had found . . . and the name Premarin: American Society for the Prevention of Cruelty to Animals website. http://www.aspca.org/fight-animal-cruelty/equine-cruelty/premarin.aspx. Accessed April 23, 2011.

Page 84 These miserable facilities: Ibid.

5. Take Two

Page 89 Here in the Hudson Valley, and all over New York state: "New York Apple Fast Facts," New York Apple Association website. http://www.nyapplecountry.com/fastfacts.htm. Accessed August 17, 2011.

Notes

Page 90 Such tail mutilation is, heartbreakingly: Susan Schoenian, "Docking, Castrating, and Debudding," University of Maryland Extension website, 2007. http://www.sheepandgoat.com/articles/castdock disb. html. Accessed May 22, 2011.

Page 91 The American Veterinary Medical Association's Animal Welfare Division: American Veterinary Medical Association's Animal Welfare Division, "Welfare Implications of Tail Docking of Lambs," American Veterinary Medical Association website, February 2010, 1–3. http://www.avma.org/issues/animal_welfare/lamb_tail_docking_bgnd.asp. Accessed April 13, 2011.

Page 91 The organization suggests using shearing: Ibid.

Page 93 And when you live with sheep and have gained their trust: Keith Kendrick et al., "Sheep Don't Forget a Face," *Nature* 414, no. 6860 (November 2001), 165.

Page 100 Carol Adams's *The Sexual Politics of Meat:* Carol J. Adams, *The Sexual Politics of Meat: A Feminist-Vegetarian Critical Theory* (New York: Continuum, 1999).

6. Dougable

Page 110 They're now friends with Mickey and Jo: F. Barbara Orlans et al., *The Human Use of Animals: Case Studies in Ethical Choice* (New York: Oxford University Press, 1998), 227–29.

7. Texas, Undercover

Page 120 As the Buddha said, "All beings tremble before violence": Judy Carman, *Peace to All Beings* (New York: Lantern, 2003), 26.

Page 121 And in the final local CBS coverage of the rescue: "Herbie the Calf Escapes Slaughter" (video), October 17, 2007. Retrieved May 23, 2011, at http://www.youtube.com/watch?v=NZoxY0dUg58.

Page 128 Fourteen *thousand*. Each *minute*: John Robbins, *The Food Revolution* (San Francisco: Conari, 2001), 214.

Notes

Page 128 That's nine billion a year in this country alone: Karen Davis, Ph.D., "Chickens," United Poultry Concerns pamphlet. http://www.upc-online .org/chickens/chickensbro.html.

Page 128 I learned that a quarter-billion baby male chicks: Foer, *Eating Animals*, 48.

Page 129 When we spread out into one of the massive cow pastures: David Degrazia, *Taking Animals Seriously: Mental Life and Moral Status* (Cambridge, England: Cambridge University Press, 1994), 283.

Page 129 When they head to slaughter: Tom Regan, *Empty Cages: Facing the Challenge of Animal Rights* (Lanham, MD: Rowman & Littlefield, 2004), 100–01.

Page 129 I learned that we force pigs into gestation crates: Jeffrey Moussaieff Masson, *The Pig Who Sang to the Moon: The Emotional World of Farm Animals* (New York: Ballantine, 2003), 39.

Page 129 "About 80 million of the 95 million hogs": Matthew Scully, *Dominion* (New York: St. Martin's, 2002), 29.

Page 134 Because of the abuse and neglect inherent: Melanie Joy, *Why We Love Dogs, Eat Pigs, and Wear Cows: An Introduction to Carnism* (San Francisco: Conari, 2010), 67.

Page 134 But no matter how sick or lame they are: United States Department of Agriculture Food Safety and Inspection Service Regulations. http://www.fsis.usda.gov/Fact_Sheets/Slaughter_Inspection_101/ index.asp. Accessed April 11, 2011.

8. My Three Hundred Chicken Roommates

Page 145 Egg farmers large and small need hens: Harvey Blatt, *America's Food: What You Don't Know About What You Eat* (Cambridge, MA: The MIT Press, 2008), 124–25.

Page 158 Merino sheep . . . are by far the most common: Regan, *Empty Cages*, 121–23.

Page 159 "Because shearers are paid by the animal, not the hour": Susie's information from "Wool," World Animal Foundation website. http://

Notes

worldanimalfoundation.homestead.com/WAF_FACT_SHEET_Wool
.pdf. Accessed May 3, 2011.

Page 159 "The shearing shed must be": Interview ibid.

Page 163 Unbelievably, "broilers" grow so quickly that they are slaughtered: "Inside the Wool Industry," People for the Ethical Treatment of Animals website. http://www.peta.org/issues/Animals-Used-for-Clothing/inside-the-wool-industry.aspx. Accessed June 5, 2011.

Page 163 These birds are kept on the floors of enormous, dark sheds: Tracye Lynn McQuirter, MPH, *By Any Greens Necessary* (Chicago: Lawrence Hill, 2010), 33. Mark H. Bernstein, *Without a Tear: Our Tragic Relationship with Animals* (Champaign: University of Illinois Press, 2004), 112.

Page 164 In the United States, ninety-five percent of hens: United Egg Producers, "United Egg Producers Animal Husbandry Guidelines for U.S. Egg Laying Flocks" (2008), 1.

Page 164 as of the end of 2008, there were 300 million hens: United States Department of Agriculture National Agriculture Statistics Service, "Chickens and Eggs" (2008), 1.

Page 164 Like any animal, chickens are highly motivated to perform natural behaviors: Sara Shields and Ian J. H. Duncan, *An HSUS Report: A Comparison of the Welfare of Hens in Battery Cages and Alternative Systems* (Washington, DC: Humane Society of the United States, 2006).

Page 164 These "spent" hens are so scrawny and bruised: "Factory Egg Production," Farm Sanctuary website. http://www.farmsanctuary.org/issues/factoryfarming/eggs. Accessed May 4, 2011.

Page 164 A layer's life, then, is several times as long as that of her broiler counterparts: "Factory Egg Production," Farm Sanctuary website. http://www.farmsanctuary.org/issues/factoryfarming/eggs. Accessed May 4, 2011.

Page 164 No wonder vegans often feel: Foer, *Eating Animals*, 60. Dawn, *Thanking the Monkey*, 169–71.

Page 165 They were valued only for their production levels: "Buckeye Egg Farm Disaster and Rescue," Farm Sanctuary website. http://www .farmsanctuary.org/rescue/rescues/past/buckeye.html. Accessed May 4, 2011.

9. Woodstock, a Wedding, and a Band of Turkeys

Page 172 Besides escaping with their lives, Boone, Alphonso, and Herschel: Ian J. H. Duncan, "A Concept of Welfare Based on Feelings," in G. John Benson and Bernard E. Rollin, eds., *The Well-Being of Farm Animals: Challenges and Solutions*, (Ames, IA: Blackwell, 2004), 96.

Page 172 Like all domesticated turkeys raised for meat: "Thanksgiving's Toll on Turkeys," Farm Sanctuary website. http://www.adoptaturkey .org/aat/issues. Accessed May 4, 2011.

Page 176 Turkeys—and commercial "broiler": "Ag Facts," Oklahoma State University Extension website. http://oklahoma4h.okstate.edu/aitc/lessons/extras/facts/turkey.html. Accessed May 4, 2011.

Page 179 "I've always viewed turkeys as smart animals": "OSU Scientist Debunks Dumb Turkey Myth," Oregon State University Extension Service website, November 19, 2003. http://extension.oregonstate.edu/ news/release/2003/11/osu-animal-scientist-debunks-dumb-turkey -myth. Accessed June 20, 2011.

Page 179 "We found that adult female birds": Quoted in David Derbyshire, "Chickens May Be Birdbrained—but They Can Still 'Feel' Each Other's Pain," *Daily Mail*, March 9, 2011. http://www.dailymail.co.uk/ sciencetech/article-1364383/Scientists-say-chickens-empathy-feel -pain.html. Accessed February 4, 2012.

Page 185 Soon after Rio's entrance came a group of hens rescued from the Buckeye Egg Farm: "Buckeye Egg Farm," Ohio History Central, http:// ohiohistorycentral.org/entry.php?rec=1672. Accessed May 28, 2011.

Page 185 The owners decided the best way to deal: "Buckeye Farm Disaster and Rescue," Farm Sanctuary website. http://www.farmsanctuary .org/rescue/rescues/past/buckeye.html. Accessed May 20, 2011.

Notes

Page 189 "When each of us comes to the end of our lives": Robbins, *The Food Revolution*, 385 (emphasis added).

Page 198 She covered everything—our chance meeting, the new EP: Fernanda Santos, "After Chance Meeting, Singer's Tribute Will Benefit an Animal Sanctuary," *New York Times*, August 4, 2009.

10. Soapbox Feet

Page 203 As Jonathan Safran Foer has written: Foer, *Eating Animals*, 258.

Page 203 "Never doubt that a *small group*: Quoted in Nancy C. Lutkehaus, *Margaret Mead: The Making of an American Icon* (Princeton, NJ: Princeton University Press, 2006), 4 (emphasis added).

Page 203 Melanie Joy, a psychologist and professor, talks about this disconnect: Joy, *Why We Love Dogs, Eat Pigs, and Wear Cows*, 29.

Pages 203–204 "We don't need meat": Ibid., 28.

Page 204 "What could cause an entire society of people . . . ?": Ibid.

Page 204 And they are "home" to ninety-nine percent of U.S. farm animals: Foer, *Eating Animals*.

Page 205 These terms aren't regulated: "How Free Is Free-Range?" "Compassion over Killing" fact sheet, http://www.cok.net/lit/freerange.php. Accessed August 23, 2011. Andrew Martin, "Meat Labels Hope to Lure the Sensitive Carnivore," *New York Times*, October 24, 2006.

Page 207 Chickens are to be consumed in quantities: Alan Scher Zagier, "Meat Industry Recruits 'Masters of Beef Advocacy' to Promote Meat Eating," *Huffington Post*, May 18, 2011. http://www.huffingtonpost.com/2011/05/18/meat-industry-recruits-ma_n_863441.html. Accessed April 23, 2011.

Page 207 The pork industry has the charming: National Pork Board website. http://www.pork4kids.com. Accessed April 23, 2011.

Page 208 But instead of having her calf's mouth on them: Karen Dawn, *Thanking the Monkey*, 167.

Notes

Page 209 Intel wrote an essay about his experience becoming vegan: Intelligent Allah, "Bread and Water Vegan," *American Vegan* 10, no. 1 (Summer 2010), 20.

Page 210 As my friend and fellow animal activist Sharon Gannon teaches: Sharon Gannon, *Yoga and Vegetarianism* (Novato, CA: Mandala, 2008), 49.

Page 210 Isaac Bashevis Singer, the great Nobel Prize–winning Yiddish writer: Will Tuttle, *The World Peace Diet* (New York: Lantern, 2005), 166.

Page 210 In his short story "The Letter Writer," he refers to farm animals: Isaac Bashevis Singer, "The Letter Writer," *The Collected Stories of Isaac Bashevis Singer* (New York: Farrar, Straus, & Giroux, 1982), 2250–76.

Page 210 I along with many others agree with Singer: Susan Ives, *Facilitator's Manual for the Class of Nonviolence* (San Antonio, TX: peaceCenter, 2007), 153.

Page 211 Charles Patterson, a Holocaust educator who came to animal issues: Charles Patterson, *Eternal Treblinka: Our Treatment of Animals and the Holocaust* (New York: Lantern, 2002).

Page 211 Patterson relates the roots of the Holocaust: Richard Schwartz, Ph.D., "Interview with Author of *Eternal Treblinka*," Jewish Vegetarians of North America website. http://www.jewishveg.com/schwartz/interview.htm. Accessed September 14, 2011.

Page 211 Many believe that examining this analogy: Ibid.

Page 211 Patterson was also influenced: Ibid.

Page 213 As Isaac Bashevis Singer said, "People often say": Ramana, *The Book of Uncommon Quips and Quotations*, 106.

Pages 213–214 You can reduce consumption simply by choosing: Meatless Monday is a project of the Monday Campaigns in association with the Johns Hopkins Bloomberg School of Public Health. http://www.meatlessmonday.com.

Page 215 According to a PCRM study, seventy-four percent: Physicians Committee for Responsible Medicine, "Congress Debates the Farm Bill," *Good Medicine* 16, no. 4 (August 2007), 1.

Notes

Page 215 "The answers . . . are matters of politics": Michael F. Jacobson, Ph.D., et al., *Six Arguments for a Greener Diet* (Washington, DC: Center for Science in the Public Interest, 2006), xiv.

Page 215 The *New York Times* food writer: Mark Bittman, "Don't End Agricultural Subsidies. Fix Them," *New York Times*, March 1, 2011.

Page 216 Bittman wants subsidies to do: Ibid.

Page 216 The other fifteen pounds are used: Frances Moore Lappé, "Like Driving a Cadillac," from *Diet for a Small Planet* (New York: Ballantine, 1982).

Page 216 And water? It takes 2,500 gallons of it to produce that: EarthSave website. http://www.earthsave.org/support/hamburgerBIG. pdf. Accessed September 13, 2011.

Page 216 Producing a calorie of meat protein: Kathy Freston, *Veganist* (New York: Weinstein, 2011), 147.

Page 217 More than sixty percent of the Amazon rainforest: http://www .physorg.com/news/2011-09-deforested-amazon-cattle.html.

Page 217 "Every second of every day": Steve Boyan, Ph.D., "How Our Food Choices Can Help Save the Environment," EarthSave website. http://www.earthsave.org/environment/foodchoices.htm. Accessed September 12, 2011.

Page 217 This in turn leads to the endangerment and extinction: Kathy Freston, "An Earth Day Reflection on the Breathtaking Effects of Cutting Down on Meat," *Huffington Post*, April 22, 2009. http://www .huffingtonpost.com/kathy-freston/an-earth-day-reflection-o_b_ 189979.html. Accessed August 23, 2011.

Page 217 "For every pound of rainforest beef": EarthSave website. http:// www.earthsave.org/support/hamburgerBIG.pdf. Accessed September 12, 2011.

Page 217 A recent United Nations report on livestock and the environment: Henning Steinfeld et al., *Livestock's Long Shadow: Environmental Issues and Options* (Rome: Food and Agriculture Organization of the UN, 2006), xx.

Notes

Page 218 Dr. Campbell's groundbreaking work *The China Study:* T. Colin Campbell, Ph.D., and Thomas M. Campbell II, *The China Study* (Dallas: BenBella, 2006).

Page 218 The results, which involved research: Ibid., 7.

Page 219 In fact, countries with the highest consumption: Ibid., 205–207.

Page 219 In all, Campbell meticulously lays out the evidence: Ibid., 7.

Page 219 Dr. Caldwell Esselstyn's twenty-year study of heart disease: Caldwell B. Esselstyn, Jr., M.D., *Prevent and Reverse Heart Disease* (New York: Avery, 2007).

Page 219 Heart disease is the leading killer in Western civilization: Ibid., 4.

Page 219 Dr. Esselstyn has had overwhelming and unequivocal success: Ibid., 95.

Page 219 These two doctors, along with many others, make it plain: The Cancer Project, Physicians Committee For Responsible Medicine: J. F. Dorgan, S. A. Hunsberger, R. P. McMahon, et al., "Diet And Sex Hormones in Girls: Findings from a Randomized Controlled Clinical Trial," *Journal of the National Cancer Institute* 95 (2003), 132–41.

Page 219 Gene Baur sums up many of these issues beautifully: Gene Baur, *Farm Sanctuary: Changing Minds About Hearts and Food* (New York: Simon & Schuster, 2008), 90.

Index

Index

Index

Index

Index